Health Risks in Today's Cosmetics

D1613772

The Handbook for A Lifetime of Healthy Skin and Hair

Nikolaus J. Smeh, M.S.

129, 117-L

ALLIANCE PUBLISHING CO.

Library of Congress Cataloging in Publication Data

Smeh, Nikolaus J.
Health Risks in Today's Cosmetics
The Handbook for a Lifetime of Healthy Skin and Hair

Includes bibliographical references and index.

1. Cosmetics. 2. Health. 3. Beauty, Personal. 4. Face-Care and Hygiene. 5. Hair-Care and Hygiene.

ISBN 0-9637755-0-2
Library of Congress Catalog Card Number: 94-071142

First Edition
Printed in the United States of America

Acknowledgements

I wish to express my sincere thanks to my son for his thorough review of the entire book, his contributions to the list of toxic substances in Appendix A, and for the graphic art portions of this publication. His efforts represent an important contribution to the book. I would also like to thank my wife for her loving support and encouragement during the writing of this book.

Please Note

This book is not intended for prescribing medication or for curing afflictions. Its purpose is not to replace the services of a physician or dermatologist but rather to serve as a reference for matters relating to healthy skin and hair. The use of any of this information for purposes of self-treatment without consulting a physician may be dangerous. Neither the publisher nor the author accept responsibility for any effects that may arise from using any type of natural treatment, or related remedy, included in this book.

Foreword

By F. Pearl McBroom, M.D. *

Nikolaus Smeh's book, Health Risks in Today's Cosmetics, provides a much needed response for information in the area of cosmetology, focusing on skin and hair renewal. Mr. Smeh suggests the need for greater supervision and research into harmful substances and carcinogens in cosmetic products. His research opens the door to more in-depth exploration in this area with potential for greater protection of the public. His research also includes the formulation of non-toxic cosmetic products, using organic and naturally-occurring substances, that represent a departure from conventional formulations. These products have produced radiant results in our office. His is an inspired goal and represents a new horizon in alternative and revitalizing measures in cosmetology. We salute you, Nikolaus Smeh, for your courage and proficiency in this creative research.

F. Pearl McBroom, M.D. is an Internist, Cardiologist, Preventive Medicine Physician in Pacific Palisades Highlands, California. Dr. McBroom is a graduate of Columbia College of Physicians & Surgeons, University of California at Los Angeles, and University of Southern California. She has done extensive research in Cardiology and is now compiling research data into chronic fatigue states and viral related disorders.

Introduction

Thousands of Americans suffer adverse effects after using off-the-shelf cosmetic products. The majority never associate burning, reddening of the skin or small pimples with a cosmetic product that they are using. Those who do seldom report it and simply discontinue using the product. Many chemicals used in cosmetics never cause signs of toxicity on the skin, but nevertheless are potent systemic toxins. The cosmetic industry has been less than enthusiastic about conducting the necessary tests to determine the short- and long-term effects of their products on consumers. Most of industry still works under the mistaken assumption that the human skin provides a sufficient barrier to irritating and toxic substances. Medical literature and hospital reports, however, have since proved them wrong.

Health Risks in Today's Cosmetics identifies the dangers of over 460 harmful ingredients used in today's cosmetic products that are sold across the United States. The medical community has provided a rich source of information about their dangers. Adverse effects of cosmetic ingredients on patients are documented by physicians and dermatologists and continuously published in medical journals and textbooks.

While pointing out dangerous substances, this handbook also identifies, whenever possible, alternative ingredients that are healthful. Many natural substances provide superior alternatives to today's toxic cosmetic ingredients. Some of them, such as oils, natural fragrances, herbs, and phospholipids, have properties that are beneficial to skin and hair. Modern science and medicine have also discovered synthetic substances that are useful and mostly harmless as cosmetic ingredients. They are either chemicals occurring in nature or are derived from natural products, such as surfactants that are made from proteins or sugars.

Cosmetic chemicals can profoundly affect the structure and health of your skin. Many how to books have been written that describe the mechanics of skin and hair care but fail to look at the effects of cosmetic ingredients. We are hopeful that this book closes that gap. Learning to avoid products that are detrimental and identifying healthful alternatives to harmful cosmetic products are keysto better living. Consumer demand for healthful alternatives to today's harmful cosmetics is the best guarantee to influence the cosmetic industry and effect the necessary changes in governmental regulation to make more healthful cosmetic products available.

Each chapter in this book stands on its own and can be read independently from the rest of the book. Certain portions of the book contain specialized information and are printed in small print to indicate that they can be skipped by the casual reader without interrupting the flow of the subject. I hope that this work will become a welcome source of information about cosmetic safety for consumers and professionals alike.

Nikolaus J. Smeh
1994

Table of Contents

Table of Figures

Table of Lists

Chapter 1

Cosmetics Today

With the advance of chemical science, a large number of synthetic chemicals have become available as raw materials for cosmetic products. Formulators of cosmetic products have an ever increasing number of possible ingredients from which to choose. The Cosmetics, Toiletry, and Fragrance Association Handbook (CTFA, 1993) lists more than 25,000 possible ingredients. Most of these have not been tested for long-term toxic and systemic effects (affecting the entire body system). Many are outright toxins or contain toxic by-products. In September 1984, the National Toxicological Program (NTP) contracted with the National Research Council (NRC) and the National Academy of Science (NAS) to study toxicity testing needs for chemical substances. The goal was to develop and validate uniformly applicable and wide-ranging criteria by which to set priorities for research of substances with potential adverse public health impact. Among the 65,725 substances considered by the NRC, 3,410 were cosmetic ingredients. The experts who participated in this vast government study concluded that "of tens of thousands of commercially important chemicals, only a few have been subjected to extensive toxicity testing and most have scarcely been tested at all."[1] There is no toxicity information available for more than 50 percent of the cosmetic ingredients used in the United States. We are now in the mid 1990s and the situation has not significantly improved.

The CTFA and the Cosmetics Industry

The cosmetics and personal care industry is represented nationally by the CTFA which provides a full range of support to meet the industry's needs and interests. The CTFA has an active membership of approximately 500. Its members include suppliers of cosmetic

---

[1] National Research Council, *Toxicity Testing: Strategies to Determine Needs and Priorities*, Washington, D.C., National Academy Press, 1984.

ingredients, manufacturers, distributors of finished personal care products, and other providers of services used in the production and marketing of cosmetic products. CTFA members market the vast majority of all personal care products sold in the United States.

The CTFA represents a powerful lobby. CTFA attorneys follow every state and federal environmental and regulatory legislation that can have an impact on the industry. They are well known in the halls of congress and in state legislatures. They have represented the interests of the cosmetic industry very well in the past. Because there is so little research into cosmetic safety, the CTFA and the cosmetic industry have been able to belittle reports of adverse effects that have been presented. When confronted by consumer organizations and congressional committees they have been able to argue successfully against increased cosmetic safety regulations because of the scarcity of toxic test studies.

The price for testing thousands of chemicals for toxicity is high. As a result, the cosmetic industry has done as little testing as possible to determine the effects of cosmetic chemicals. The cosmetic industry has voluntarily established a limited testing program for cosmetic ingredients through the Cosmetic Ingredient Review (CIR) which was established in 1976 by the CTFA. Their reports are published in the Journal of the American College of Toxicology. So far they have reviewed and issued reports on 379 ingredients. The most recent additions to the list of unsafe chemicals used in cosmetic products include: chloracetamide (all uses), formaldehyde (unsafe for use in aerosol products), HC Blue No. 1 (all uses), hydroquinone (unsafe for use in leave-on products), p-hydroxyanisole (all uses), methenamine (unsafe for use in aerosol products), 4-methoxy-m-phenylenediamine (all uses), and monoethanolamine (unsafe for use in leave-on products). Over 3,000 of the 3,410 NCR-identified cosmetic chemicals (with potential adverse health impact) remain untested. New cosmetic chemicals and manufacturing processes (that can produce hazardous by-products) are coming into the market almost daily. In the meantime, the U.S. population is exposed to potential cancer-causing and mutagenic chemicals on a daily basis.

The FDA

The U.S. Department of Health and Human Services, Food and Drug Administration (FDA) is responsible for regulating all matters related to food, drugs, and cosmetics. The FDA has an annual budget of $800 million (with over 9,000 full-time employees), but spends less than one percent of its budget on regulatory supervision of the cosmetic industry — an industry which produces over 20,000 products with an estimated annual volume of about 18 billion dollars. Approximately 400 inspectors must cover the national and international multibillion dollar food and cosmetic industries, and about 60 toxicologists are responsible for evaluating all cosmetic and food products.

Scientists in FDA laboratories survey and test cosmetic products for toxic substances, and identify cosmetic materials that can cause adverse effects. They also initiate research to support additional cosmetic regulations to the Code of Federal Regulations (CFR). The FDA sometimes seeks voluntary compliance by the Cosmetic Industry with proposed legislation during the sometimes lengthy process before such regulations become law. Two of the most recent examples are in Proposed 21 CFR §700.20 that deals with certain hormones as ingredients in cosmetic products, and in Proposed 21 CFR §700.35 that will regulate the use of sunscreens and claims by manufacturers of sunscreen products. In the dynamic cosmetic industry new products accompanied by new claims appear very frequently and need to be verified and tested. One of the latest fads is the use of alpha hydroxy acids. The agency has just completed an investigation of over forty alpha hydroxy acids products and found the ingredients resorcinol (which causes discoloration and dermatitis) and phenol (which causes depigmentation and contact urticaria) in the preparations. A final report on these types of ingredients and recommendations for use will be available by the end of 1994.

The FDA and consumer organizations have fought long and hard in the attempt to influence legislators to remove toxic substances from the cosmetic market as soon as test results are available. Among those that have successfully been removed in the recent past are chlorofluorocarbon, methylene chloride, acetylethyltetramethyltetralin, and certain tar colors.

The CFR has several laws that apply to the cosmetics and hair care industry. The law defines cosmetics as articles intended to be applied to the human body for "cleansing, beautifying, promoting attractiveness or altering the appearance" without affecting the body's structure or function.[2] Cosmetic products intended to affect the structure or functions of the human body must meet the more stringent regulations imposed on the drug industry. The following paragraphs describe the main provisions of the law that deal with Adulterated and Misbranded Cosmetics, Cosmetic Safety, Cosmetic Labeling and Declaration of Ingredients.

Adulterated or Misbranded Cosmetics Regulation

A cosmetic product is considered adulterated if it contains one or more substances that are harmful to consumers under customary use. Clinical studies conducted over the past two decades reveal that many frequently used ingredients in cosmetic products are harmful. As a result, most of the products sold in the United States contain one or two of these substances and should be taken off the market under this provision. In addition, many otherwise harmless ingredients can contain very toxic byproducts or contaminants that never appear on the label. Examples of these substances are ethylene oxide (a potent toxin) and amines that can form carcinogenic nitrosamines in the skin. These can also be considered adulteration and the products should be banned from the market place.

A cosmetic product is considered as misbranded if its labeling is false or misleading, if it doesn't have the required labeling information, or is made or filled in a deceptive manner. Any claims by a manufacturers that the product changes the structure of the skin fall into this

---

[2] U.S. Department of Health and Human Services, *Federal Food, Drug, and Cosmetic Act, as Amended, and Related Laws*, Sec. 201(g)(1), Washington, D.C., 1989.

category. Examples of unacceptable language are statements including claims to stop, reverse, or reduce the signs of aging, as well as statements implying protection against formation of cancer or other skin diseases. Another example is the suggestion by many manufacturers that the use of animal collagen and elastin, or cells from human fetuses, in skin products can somehow replace aging skin cells. There is absolutely no proof of this and all such products should be removed from the market.

Cosmetic Safety Regulation

Although the Federal Drug and Cosmetic Act does not require cosmetic manufacturers or marketers to test their product for safety, the FDA strongly urges cosmetic manufacturers to conduct whatever toxicological or other tests that are appropriate to prove the safety of their products. A 1993 FDA market survey found levels of the highly toxic 1,4-dioxane in 27 out of 30 children's shampoo and bubble bath products analyzed, as well as in all of the 54 ethoxylated cosmetic raw materials tested. Except for a few prohibited ingredients, a cosmetic manufacturer may use essentially any raw material as a cosmetic ingredient and market the product without approval. The FDA requires that cosmetic manufacturers put a label on untested products that are not proven to be safe. Most manufacturers have not complied because of the absence of a Congressional law mandating such action.

Cosmetic Labeling and Declaration of Ingredient Regulation

Two of the most beneficial parts of the Federal Drug and Cosmetic Act to the consumer are the provisions for Cosmetic Labeling and Declaration of Ingredients. Under this provision, all retail products must contain a list of ingredients in descending order of predominance. Unfortunately, only those with chemistry, physics, and medical backgrounds can understand the nature of most ingredients listed. This book identifies many harmful substances which will help you to avoid potentially harmful ingredients. (See Appendix A which lists several hundred harmful ingredients commonly found in cosmetic products.)

Cosmetic products that are not distributed through retail channels are exempt from the above requirement. Thus, manufacturers of hair preparations, makeup products, and skin care products that are used by professionals in beauty salons are exempt from labeling and declaring of ingredients. This places the customer at risk by being unable to inspect product ingredients. Few cosmetic professionals are aware of the potentially dangerous chemicals used in their work place. In a study conducted by the University of California of more than 58,000 hairdressers, manicurists, and cosmetologists revealed that they developed multiple myeloma (cancer) at four times the rate of the general population. This is believed to be due to their work environment.[3]

Studies on Harmful Cosmetic Ingredients

To this day, thousands of unsuspecting people use off-the-shelf cosmetic products and suffer adverse effects. Many simply stop the use of a particular product when developing skin problems and never see a doctor. A large number, especially those who develop more severe problems, see a dermatologist, who, after many patch tests, may find the chemical that causes the problem and link it to a cream, lotion, or hair care product. If there is a frequent recurrence of skin problems from a particular chemical, doctors publish their findings in the professional literature. When it became apparent to professionals in the 1970s that frequent occurrences of skin diseases, including cancer, could be traced to chemicals in cosmetic products, many ad- hoc study groups formed all over the world to investigate. Soon text books appeared at medical schools that were dedicated to cosmetics and dermatology. All this information can be accessed today on computers and with the advances of computer and storage technology it is possible to capture all this research into large databases. Thousands of professional medical articles are now available on the adverse effects from today's cosmetics. These articles represent the work of hundreds of medical doctors as they have documented and published actual case histories of patients with skin problems caused by cosmetic products. The references in this book are representative of the wealth of materials available on this subject and span a period of over fifteen years. Almost all problem chemicals reported during this period in the medical literature can still be found in cosmetic products in the U.S. today.

Summary of Findings

My recent survey of today's cosmetic products revealed surprising results. Over eighty percent of the products on the market today contain one or more ingredients that are documented to cause adverse reactions in humans and animals. Professionals agree that only a few incidents are reported since affected consumers simply discontinue using the product. Many resulting systemic effects are unknown and remain undiagnosed and an unsuspecting population remains unwarned.

The question naturally arises: Why do manufacturers continue to use chemicals with known adverse effects in cosmetic products? There is no simple answer to this question.

---

[3]   Ames, Bruce N. Dr., Research on mutagenicity of hair dyes, Biochemistry Department of the University of California at Berkeley, 1978 Congressional Hearings.

Some reasons may include the following:

- a lack of consumer awareness.
- a lack of sufficient industrial regulations and enforcement of the existing laws by the government.
- a lack of sufficient testing of chemicals used in cosmetics for long-term effects on humans.

- convenience of manufacturing products with long shelf life (requiring large amounts of toxic preservatives).
- superior formulation properties of certain synthetic chemicals.
- unwillingness by many manufacturers to pay higher prices for more refined ingredients.
- adherence to an "acceptable risk" doctrine (even though a small number of individuals do experience severe adverse reactions, they represent an acceptable risk to the manufacturers since most of the victims just discontinue use after having an adverse reaction).

Protecting Yourself from Harmful Cosmetic Products

There is a simple way to protect yourself from harmful cosmetic products. As a result of the Labeling and Declaration of Ingredients provision in the Federal Drug and Cosmetic Act, all manufacturers are required to list ingredients on the label. Once harmful ingredients have been identified, this listing provides an easy way for you to avoid using harmful products. If enough consumers compare ingredient labels with lists of known harmful chemicals and refuse to buy harmful products, they will eventually disappear from the marketplace.

In the past, lists of harmful cosmetic ingredients were published only in textbooks for medical doctors and toxicologists. This publication makes such a list available for the first time to the general public. Appendix A contains a listing of over 450 cosmetic chemicals with known harmful effects to your skin or body as identified by the medical community. To benefit from this information you need to read the label on the cosmetic products you are using today and compare the ingredients with those listed in Appendix A.

Healthy and Natural Alternatives

A natural outgrowth of this study was an effort to determine the feasibility of formulating skin and hair care products free of any harmful ingredients. After eliminating all harmful substances found in the medical literature, the remaining, mostly natural, ingredients were evaluated from a dermatological perspective (concerning skin compatibility) and investigated for possible toxic contamination or unwanted byproducts resulting from the manufacturing process. Those substances which passed this initial screening were then analyzed by cosmetic formulators to determine their suitability for use in cosmetic products. After extensive laboratory studies and the cooperation by manufacturers of cosmetic raw materials, it was found that it is feasible to manufacture healthful cosmetic products that they are superior in quality to their unhealthful counterparts and that there are enough nonirritating and nontoxic ingredients available today to allow the formulation of most cosmetic products on the market. These studies also revealed that some natural skin and hair care ingredients, although more expensive, are vastly superior to their synthetic counterparts. The remainder of this book identifies both healthful and harmful cosmetic ingredients.

Chapter 2

Basic Cosmetic Materials

Cosmetics are complicated mixtures of chemical compounds. The CTFA *International Buyer's Guide* lists over 25,000 ingredients available to cosmetic formulators from various manufacturers of raw materials. Any one of these ingredients can be chosen to formulate a given moisturizing cream, lotion or other cosmetic product. This abundant availability of ingredients has created the opportunity for endless varieties in cosmetic formulations. Product appearance, shelf life, and cost of materials are main factors in choosing ingredients. Raw materials must be of predictable composition to ensure successful formulation each time the product is manufactured. Synthetic raw materials fit these requirements and are the main choice of manufacturers.

The mistaken assumption that the skin forms an impenetrable barrier to chemical substances has led the industry to neglect sufficient testing of synthetic ingredients for irritating, mutagenic, toxic, and carcinogenic properties. The permeability (see glossary) of the skin to chemicals has been known for over two decades. However, no major effort is underway by government or industry to require sufficient long term toxicological testing of cosmetic materials. It is a tragedy that U.S. consumers are involuntarily used as test subjects for ingredients and that thousands must suffer adverse reactions before offending substances are taken off the market.

Before 1979 it was difficult to obtain information on the ingredients used in cosmetic formulations. The introduction of mandatory ingredient labeling in the U.S. (since April 15, 1977) has been a great improvement. The interested consumer can avoid using products containing ingredients with known adverse effects by checking product labels. The dermatologist and the consumer are now in a better position to detect adverse reactions through patch testing since each ingredient listed can now be tested separately.

No completely natural cosmetic products are available on the commercial market. One reason is that commercial products are formulated for a shelf life of about three years, and as a result must contain sufficient amounts of preservatives to prevent spoiling. Natural cosmetics preserved with natural anti-bacterial and anti-oxidants are unable to compete with this shelf life requirement. There are a few companies in the U.S. who manufacture cosmetic products using materials derived from natural sources only, except for preservatives. Products without preservatives, by necessity, must have a stated limited shelf life (much like food products in the supermarket) and must be refrigerated.

There is a wealth of information and practical knowledge available about natural products because mankind has used them for thousands of years. There are advantages in using food grade materials for cosmetics because they are under much greater scrutiny by the FDA than are synthetic cosmetic raw materials. This includes using food-grade fats and oils that are, with water, major ingredients in creams and lotions as well other biological products, like herbs, gums, and essential oils.. However, there are some natural materials that are also harmful. This is mostly true for some plant materials and otherwise harmless color pigments that may be contaminated by heavy metal salts. Talcum powder, for instance, can be contaminated by asbestos, a known carcinogen. [4]

Modern chemistry has been successful in synthesizing many materials occurring in nature. It has also been successful in producing derivatives of natural products for the food industry, like margarine (hydrogenated natural oils), and emulsifiers which are used in a variety of edible products, from baked goods to mayonnaise and ice cream. One problem with using synthetic materials are the contaminants that are created during the manufacturing process. These can be highly toxic in very small amounts. They are so potent that their content in cosmetic raw materials is measured in parts per million (ppm). One ppm, for instance, represents a concentration of one thousandth of a gram of contaminant in one kilogram of material. Recent advances in chemical analysis have made it possible to easily detect such small amounts of highly toxic substances. The medical and chemical literature is full of reports on how to detect such minute amounts of harmful chemicals (like ethylene oxide, dioxane, and nitrosamines) in food and cosmetics. Synthetic fragrances, emulsifiers, solubilizers, and surfactants are among the prime suspects for contamination.

In recommending healthy cosmetic ingredients I give natural products first choice, and synthesized versions of natural products second choice. An example would be natural Vitamin C from Rose Hips compared to synthetic Vitamin C which is chemically equivalent. Only if these materials are not available do I recommend substances that are chemically derived from natural products, like surfactants containing amino acids (glycine) or sucrose. Only as last resort should synthetic ingredients be considered, and only if they have been proven harmless and have been found free of contaminants.

The human skin protects itself from the outside world by producing a natural skin cream that consists mainly of sebum, phospholipids, cholesterol, and water. It is well known that water and oil do not mix no matter how hard one tries. Nature has found a way to accomplish the mixing of oil and water by introducing substances called emulsifiers, which function as intermediaries between oil and water. They are able to form mixtures consisting of microscopic droplets of oil dispersed in water. While water and oil appear transparent, emulsions are usually white or opaque because of the scattering of light on the microscopic oil droplets. Natural examples of emulsions are milk and mayonnaise. In the following two sections I will describe the two main ingredients of creams and lotions besides water, emollients (oils) and emulsifiers.

[4] Blount A.M., Geology Department, Amphibole (asbestos) content of cosmetic and pharmaceutical talcs, Rutgers University, Newark, NJ 07102, *Environ. Health Perspect.* 1991 Aug, 94, 225-30.

Emollients

Cosmetic creams and lotions are formulated to imitate the natural protective layer of the skin and consist of manmade emulsions. The basic ingredients are always water, emollients (oils, fats, lipids) and emulsifiers. There are a wealth of natural and synthetic emollients available for cosmetic products. In this section you will find evidence that the benefits of using natural emollients in cosmetic products far outweigh those using their synthetic counterparts.

A small amount of conceptual knowledge is necessary to understand the phenomenon of oils, emulsions, soaps and detergents. This knowledge will also help you understand the newest concept in skin care — the use of liposomes. Natural oils and fats are complex compounds called triglycerides. Each molecule is formed from glycerin and three fatty acids. If you could see a fatty acid molecule it would look like a round match, a spherical head and a long tail. The long tail is composed of a chain of carbon and hydrogen atoms and is of

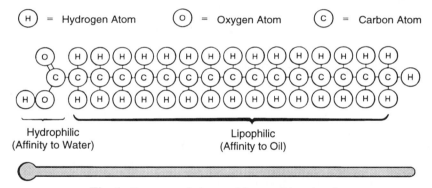

Fig. 1 *Conceptual shape of fatty acid molecule*

varying length depending on the number of carbon atoms in the chain. The head is made up of two oxygen and one hydrogen atom bonded to the first carbon atom on the chain as shown in Figure 1. The long tail of this molecule is lipophilic which means having an affinity for oil. The head at the hydrogen-oxygen (OH-) position is hydrophilic which means having an affinity for water.

The second component of an oil is glycerin, which is an alcohol that has three hydrogen-oxygen group (OH-) locations on its molecule where hydrophilic molecules can readily attach. These hydrogen-oxygen groups are responsible for the great affinity of glycerine to water. The hydrophilic portions of three fatty acids can attach at these locations under special circumstances. Thus, plants and animals manufacture oils and fat by joining glycerin and three fatty acids as part of the metabolic process. A simplified presentation of an oil molecule, or triglyceride, is shown in Figure 2. After this synthesis is completed, no more OH- locations with affinity to water remain on the molecule. They become lipophilic compounds that are immiscible with water, as common oils are. All oils and fats in the plant and animal world are mixtures of triglycerides with different fatty acid contents.

Fatty acid compounds play a large role in the cosmetic industry as emollients and in the chemical synthesis of emulsifiers and detergents. Since you will encounter them when checking the labels of cosmetic products, I have included a detailed description of several natural and synthetic emollients in this section. Naturally occurring oils, fats, and waxes are all mixtures of various triglycerides. Since the fatty acid mix may vary widely depending on growth season and location, each natural oil must be specially formulated for a particular product. Many fatty acids, fatty alcohols and esters, and alkoxylated compounds can be synthesized today and are preferred by cosmetic formulators as emollients to

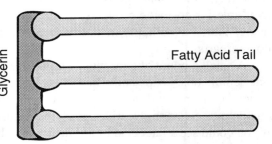

Fig. 2 *Conceptual shape of oil molecule (triglyceride)*

natural products because of the predictable outcome of formulations. Unfortunately, synthesis can introduce unwanted by-products and contaminants. It is safer to use natural emollients for skin creams and lotions although they may be more expensive than their synthetic counterparts and more difficult to formulate into products.

Natural oils should be cold pressed to yield the added benefits of valuable substances like vitamins, essential fatty acids, unsaturated oils, and ingredients called unsaponifiables (compounds that cannot be converted to soaps, or saponified, upon addition of alkali), because they are all valuable skin conditioning agents. Of special value are oils that contain essential fatty acids because these cannot be synthesized in the human body. The most important are the linoleic, linolenic, and arachidonic acids. They are also known as Vitamin F and are effective in treating skin conditions like dermatitis, and are building blocks for a class of important regulating substances in the human body called prostaglandins. For example, Prostaglandin E1 is effective in very small amounts to liberate fat deposits in human tissues. A deficiency of these essential fatty acids in the human diet can also cause hair loss. Natural oils rich in unsaturated fatty acids are safflower oil (70%), soybean oil (61%), sunflower oil (60%), borage oil (55%), wheat germ oil (54%), corn germ oil (54%), sesame oil (46%), almond oil (25%), olive oil (16%) and avocado oil (16%). A summary of the average fatty acid content of these and some additional oils and fats is given in Table 1.

Table 1 Average Fatty Acid Content of Fats and Oils in Percent

Fatty Acid	lauric	myristic	palmitic	palmitoleic	stearic	oleic	linoleic	linolenic	arachidic	sterolins
C Atoms / un-saturated chains	12/0	14/0	16/0	16/1	18/0	18/1	18/2	18/3	20/0	
Fats										
Almond Oil			7		2	64	24	trace		1
Apricot Oil			3		1	60	30	trace		
Avocado Oil		1	8	3	2	68	15	2		6
Borage Oil			8		8	26	35	19		trace
Cocoa Butter	44	18	11		6	7	2			
Maize Oil			14		4	29	52		trace	6
Cotton Oil		trace	19			33	39		1	(*)
Jojoba Oil	Jojoba Oil is a wax with multiple unsaturated carbon chains from C40 to C44									
Olive Oil			17	2	2	60	16	2		1
Palmkernel Oil	51	17	8		2	13	2			
Safflower Oil			6		3	12	70	1	1	
Sesame Oil			10	trace	5	42	41	1		1
Shea Butter	4		trace		25	60				10
Soya Oil			9		4	25	51	7	2	1
Sunflower Oil			9		4	28	58			trace
Wheatgerm Oil			14		3	27	43	10	1	trace
Animal fats										
Butter	4	12	29	5	11	25		2	2	2
Lard		3	26	6	17	43	4			
Tallow		3	24	3	18	42	9		2	

(*) The unrefined oil contains in excess of 10 % sterolins

Unsaponifiables contained in natural oils consist mainly of a group of compounds called plant steroids or sterolins. They have many positive attributes especially useful for skin care. Among the most important are their ability to soften the skin, have a superior moisturizing effect on the upper layer of skin, and have a positive effect in the treatment of scars. The sterolins in avocado oil have been found to help diminish age spots. The highest content of these substances can be found in sheabutter (3.5-11%), avocado oil (2-6%), sesame oil (1-1.5%), soybean oil (0.5-1.5%), with smaller amounts found in linseed oil, olive oil, and peanut oil.

Processing of Plant Oils and Fats

There are more than 150 different plant oils that can be produced, but only a few have commercial value for the food and cosmetic industry. In their natural state they contain a variety of substances that can be beneficial to the skin. Modern processing methods almost completely remove these natural compounds to obtain a better color, odor, or increased shelf life of the finished product. The two main processing methods used to produce oil from plant materials are hydraulic pressing (cold or hot), and extraction by organic solvents (such as hexane). Only cold pressing yields an acceptable oil for cosmetics since it seldom needs further processing and yields a pure product.

Hot-pressed and extracted oils require subsequent refining which results in the loss of many valuable ingredients. Depending on the number of undesirable components to be removed, many of which are beneficial for skin care, the refining process may consist of the following steps:

— De-sliming: Natural oil is mixed with hot water to which phosphoric acid or citric acid is added. The phospholipids (valuable components for skin care) are transformed into an insoluble form and separated by centrifugation

— De-acidification: Free fatty acids are bound (saponified) by an alkaline solution or removed by vacuum distillation.

— Bleaching: The de-acidified oil is bleached by a treatment at 90° C with Fuller's earth (adsorbent clay) and then filtered.

— Homogenization: Undesirable odor and taste compounds are removed by hot steam and heating the oil to 150° C (327° F) for a prolonged period.

In the case of extracted and hot-pressed oils the result is a truly refined product, void of most vitamins and other beneficial compounds for skin care.

The following is a brief description of some important plant oils and fats that can be used in cosmetics.

Natural Emollients

Almond oil (prunus amygdalus): The almond tree is cultivated in Southern Europe, the Mediterranean countries and in California. The kernel contains up to 60 percent of this high priced oil that consists mainly of oleic acid, essential unsaturated fatty acids (about 25%), sterolins (from 0.5 to 1.0%) and vitamin E (about 10 International Units [IU] per ounce). Almond oil was highly valued by the Egyptians for cosmetic purposes. It is known for its mildness, has excellent shelf life and imparts a soft feel to creams and lotions.

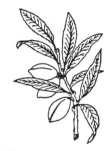

Fig. 3 *Almond (prunus amygdalus)*

Apricot kernel oil (prunus armeniaca): The apricot tree is cultivated throughout the northern hemisphere. The kernel contains up to 45 percent oil that is very similar to almond oil except for a higher unsaturated essential fatty acid content of 30 percent. It also gives creams and lotions a soft feel and spreadability, but is less stable than almond oil.

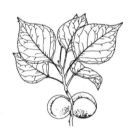

Fig. 4 *Apricot (prunus armeniaca)*

Avocado oil (persea americana): Avocado oil is a very stable oil that contains more than 20 percent essential unsaturated fatty acids. Almost all vitamins can be found in the unprocessed oil in significant amounts and also a small amount of lecithin. The content of unsaponifiables (sterolins) is significant. Unfortunately, part of them are frequently removed and sold separately as a high-priced cosmetic raw material. The age of skin is partly determined by its content of soluble collagen. A recent study found that treatment with avocado oil significantly increases the water soluble collagen content in the dermis. It is, therefore, a highly valued oil for creams and lotions, but is very expensive. The skin compatibility of avocado oil is excellent and it also has very good spreadability. In addition, it somewhat protects the skin from ultraviolet rays.

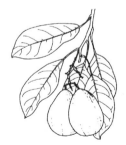

Fig. 5 *Avocado (persea americana)*

Borago Oil (borago officinalis): Borago oil is obtained from the seed of borago officinalis, an annual plant that grows abundantly in the Mediterranean region as well as Central Europe and Asia.

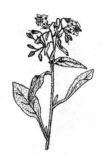

Fig. 6 *Borago (borago officinalis)*

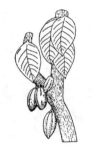

Fig. 7 *Coca tree (theobroma cacao)*

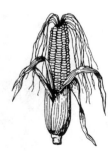

Fig. 8 *Corn (zea mays)*

There has been great interest in recent years in growing this plant commercially in the U.S. because of the high Gamma-Linolenic Acid (GLA) content in its oil. GLA is necessary for the synthesis of prostaglandin, which has important functions in the human body and especially for the skin. The only other commercial source for GLA is evening primrose oil (enothera biennis). Borago oil has also the highest known content of other essential unsaturated fatty acids that are valuable skin conditioning agents and are also used for medicinal purposes. Essential fatty acids seem to regulate the hydration of the skin and act as natural humectants. The oil also appears promising in treating atopic eczema. Borage oil is expensive and is mainly used as emollient for anti-aging creams and lotions and for medicinal purposes.

Cocoa butter (theobroma cacao): The cocoa tree is native to the Amazon valley but is extensively cultivated in almost all tropical countries. Cocoa butter is obtained from the seeds (which are commonly known as beans) and is a by-product from the manufacture of cocoa and chocolate. It is solid at room temperature and contains about 5 IU of vitamin E per ounce. Cocoa butter is mainly used as a thickening agent in cosmetics. It can be used with almost all natural oils and is well absorbed by the skin. Because it leaves a sheen on the skin, its main application is for night creams and lotions. Cocoa butter can promote acne and is not recommended for oily skin.

Corn oil (zea mays): The United States is the largest producer of corn in the world. As the corn is processed into meal, starch, glucose and other products, the germ must be mechanically removed. The germ is the valued byproduct used for the production of corn oil. Corn oil is very rich in unsaturated fatty acids (58%) and contains up to 2 percent of plant sterolins that are valuable for cosmetic purposes. Cold pressed corn oils contain up to 25 IU of vitamin E per ounce and are well suited for use as inexpensive emollients for creams and lotions.

Cottonseed oil (gossypium hirsutum, barbadense): Wild species of cotton grow in the tropical regions in both hemispheres in the form of small trees. From these species, hundreds of cultivated varieties have been developed that are grown as an annual crop. The oil-carrying parts are the seeds that are embedded in the cotton fiber. Cottonseed oil goes through a long refining process before it becomes suitable for consumption and cosmetic purposes. The refined oil still contains about 20 IU of vitamin E per ounce and has a high content (39%) of essential unsaturated fatty acids that are important for skin care. Mixed with other oils, it can be used as cosmetic emollient and yields a soft, easily spreadable cream.

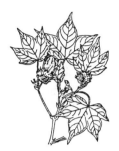

Fig. 9 *Cotton (gossypium hirsutum)*

Jojoba oil (simmondsis chinensis): The jojoba tree is cultivated in California, Arizona, Mexico and Israel. It grows well in the arid areas where no other cash crop will grow. Jojoba oil is produced from the fruits of the jojoba tree by cold pressing. Chemically speaking, it is not an oil but a wax with long unsaturated carbon chains. The importance of jojoba oil for the cosmetic industry stems from its chemical similarity to sperm whale oil or spermaceti oil. Spermaceti was a valued ingredient in cosmetic creams. Its widespread use contributed to the extinction of sperm whales and was outlawed many years ago. Spermaceti has been replaced in most cases with synthetic products, like cetyl alcohol, that cause adverse skin reactions. Jojoba oil is the ideal replacement for the now-unavailable spermaceti. It is a natural, stable compound that has superior properties that leave the skin soft, supple, and smooth. It heals acne prone skin and acts as a sunscreen. Therefore, it more than replaces spermaceti oil. Its wider use is only inhibited by its high price.

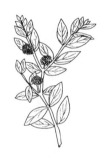

Fig. 10 *Jojoba (simmondsis chinensis)*

Olive oil (olea europaea): The olive tree is an evergreen, native to the Mediterranean area but widely grown in tropical areas and warm climates. Olive oil is one of the most important and ancient oils, and is the most widely used oil in the countries bordering the Mediterranean. The oil is obtained by crushing and pressing the fruit which produces the characteristic color and flavor. Despite

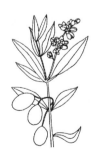

Fig. 11 *Olive (olea europaea)*

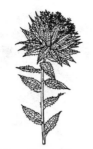

Fig. 12 *Safflower (carthamus tinctorius)*

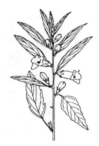

Fig. 13 *Sesame (sesamum indicum)*

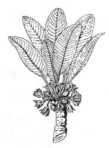

Fig. 14 *Shea tree (butyrospermum parkii)*

its odor, it has been used since time immemorial for cosmetic purposes. It has been recently shown to promote acne (comedogenic) and therefore is not recommended as an emollient for creams and lotions.

Safflower oil (carthamus tinctorius): Safflower is an annual plant native to the Mediterranean countries and is cultivated in Europe and in the United States. It has been known since ancient times but has just recently obtained commercial importance as an edible oil. The oil is obtained by pressing or solvent extraction. Safflower oil has one of the highest linoleic acid content of all known oils. This unsaturated fatty acid compound gives the oil a superior skin compatibility and deep moisturizing capability since the moisture content of the skin is proportional to the content of essential unsaturated fatty acids. It is well suited for the production of creams, lotions and bath oils.

Sesame oil (sesamum indicum): Sesame oil has been known for thousands of years. It is produced from the tiny seeds of the sesame plant that is grown mainly in China and India. The cold pressed crude oil is of high quality and valued as one of the best salad oils. It is used in cosmetics because of its content of sterolins which are valuable moisturizers and skin conditioning agents.

Shea butter (butyrospermum parkii): The plant butter is produced from the nuts of a large tree, called bassia parkii, which is abundant on the West Coast of Africa. It is used as food and for body care by the natives. It is used in cosmetics as a thickening agent for creams and lotions and imparts superior softness to the skin because of its high content of unsaponifiables and cinnamic esters, which have antimicrobial and moisturizing properties. In addition, shea butter contains vitamins and allantoin that gives it healing properties.

Soybean oil (soya max): The soybean has been cultivated since prehistoric times in the Orient because of its protein, oil, and lecithin content. Today, soybean oil is the most important oil produced in the United States. It is produced from the seed of the soybean by pressing or solvent extraction. The crude oil must be refined to remove protein and lecithin which form a valuable byproduct of the soy oil production. Most of the lecithin (phospholipids) used in cosmetics today is derived from soybeans. Soybean oil is very high in unsaturated fatty acid compounds and has a high vitamin E content of 30 IU per ounce (which is also the recommended daily requirement [RDR] for an adult person). All these properties, together with an up to two percent content of skin softening sterolins, make the soybean oil a valued emollient for all applications. Its somewhat darker color may give creams and lotion a slight coloring.

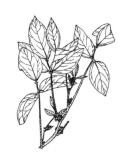

Fig. 15 *Soja (soya max)*

Wheatgerm oil (triticum): Although wheat germ oil is normally not used as emollient for creams and lotions it is mentioned because of its high content of several important active ingredients for skin care. Wheatgerm oil has the highest vitamin E content of any oil (250 IU per ounce). In addition it contains provitamin A and D, lecithin, and a high content of unsaturated fatty acid compounds. Creams and lotions manufactured with wheatgerm oil have a yellowish color and have the characteristic smell of wheat that cannot easily be masked by the addition of masking fragrances.

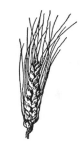

Fig. 16 *Wheat (triticum)*

Synthetic Emollients

Synthetic emollients are by far the most popular choice for cosmetic manufacturers and formulators. Of the 500 most popular emollients used in today's cosmetic products only about 8 percent are of natural origin. Of the remaining 92 percent of synthetic emollients over half have been cited in the medical literature for having caused adverse skin reactions in some section of the population. The most important groups of synthetic chemicals used as emollients are briefly described below:

Alkoxylated Carboxylic Acids: Chemically, these emollients are made by combining polyethylene glycol (an alcohol) with one of the many fatty acids to form an ester or ether. On the label of cosmetic products they are listed as PEG-n with the name of a fatty acid salt added, like PEG-8 Laurate (lauric acid compound). All chemicals with the designation PEG may contain some amount of the toxic chemical 1,4-dioxane (Ref. 150) as a manufacturing by-product. A recent analysis of a cross section of cosmetic products confirms the continuing problem with dioxane (Ref. 179).

Esters: Esters are compounds formed between acids and alcohols. Synthetic esters can be formed by combining any type of alcohol with an organic or inorganic acid. Thus, the number of synthetic esters that are used in cosmetics as emollients is very large. On ingredient labels they are identified by the name of the alcohol and the acid used like Amyl Acetate (amyl alcohol and acetic acid), or Propylene Glycol Laurate. Chemical compounds containing the following alcohols have been shown to cause allergies and dermatitis: benzyl-, butyl-, cetearyl-, cetyl-, decyl-, dimethyl-, ethyl-, glyceryl-, isopropyl-, lanolin-, methyl-, myristyl-, polyethylene-, polypropylene-, propyl-, propylene-, and stearyl alcohols. In addition, all compound names containing the designation PEG and -eth (like laureth), can contain appreciable amounts of the carcinogen 1,4-dioxane.

Fatty Alcohols: Fatty alcohols are higher molecular weight non-volatile alcohols that are used as reactive components for the synthesis of a variety of cosmetic chemicals. By themselves, they are used as emollients as well as co-emulsifiers to increase viscosity of cosmetic products. They always contain the name "alcohol" on the ingredient label. Both of the two most popular fatty alcohols used as emollients, cetyl alcohol and cetearyl alcohol, have been shown to cause contact eczema (see Ref. 100, 134).

Glyceryl Esters and Derivatives: Plant oils are natural esters formed by glycerine (an alcohol) and fatty acids and are called triglycerides. They are natural mixtures of many different fatty acid compounds and are used as raw materials to produce glycerine and fatty acids. Although the original oil or fat may not be suitable for cosmetics (fish oil, lard, etc.) the fatty acids can be separated and re-combined with glycerine or other alcohols through synthesis to form a more usable product. They are listed on the ingredient label as "glyceryl" with the name of the fatty acid added, like glyceryl oleate. Some are close to compounds found in nature but have been found to cause dermatitis, like glyceryl oleate and glyceryl stearate (see Appendix A). Those products using polyethylene glycol (PEG) for the synthesis suffer from the same problem of 1,4-dioxane contamination as mentioned previously. Another group of modified natural fats and oils is obtained by hydrogenation. This process chemically alters the fatty acid carbon chains and solidifies the compound. Unfortunately, all the unsaturated fatty acids that are valuable components for skin care are eliminated in this process.

Hydrocarbons: Hydrocarbons are generally derived from petro chemicals. Typically they are the higher boiling petroleum distillates like mineral oils and paraffins and find extensive applications as lubricants (motor oils). In their more refined form they are widely used as emollients in cosmetics creams and lotions (especially suntan lotions) because of their inertness and non-volatility. Recently it has been found that even the highly refined hydrocarbons used for cosmetic products can contain carcinogenic and mutagenic Polycyclic Aromatic Hydrocarbons (PAH) and the carcinogen Anthanthrene (Ref. 95). In addition, mineral oil and petrolatum can cause chemically induced acne (Ref. 130).

Lanolin and Lanolin Derivatives: Also known as wool wax, lanolin is a complex mixture of high molecular esters of fatty acids. It is an important commercial source for sterols and its derivatives and are widely used in cosmetics for skin and hair care. Lanolin has been used in cosmetic preparations since the time of the Egyptian Empire. Recently, a number of cases of lanolin sensitivity and contact dermatitis have been reported in the literature (Ref. 17, 82, 120).

Emulsifiers

An emulsifier is a chemical compound that is used to join oil and water to form a stable mixture called emulsion. Each emulsifier molecule has the unique property to attract both water and oil at the same time at different sites of its structure (See Figure 17). Emulsifiers based on fatty acids and glycerin from plant and animal fats have a similar conceptual structure as shown in Fig. 2 (chapter on emollients), except for one difference: one or two of the fatty acid chains have been chemically removed leaving one or two hydrophilic sites vacant on the glycerine molecule. The resulting compounds are called diglycerides and

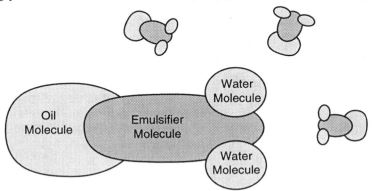

Fig. 17 *Conceptual shape of molecular element of emulsion*

monoglycerides respectively and their conceptual shape is given in Figure 18. The one or two locations on the glycerin molecule without an attached fatty acid have a high affinity to water

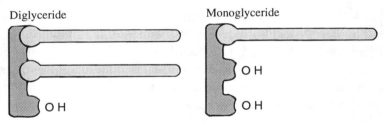

Fig. 18 *Conceptual shape of emulsifier molecules (glycerides)*

while the remaining fatty acid tails attract oily compounds. Thus, the emulsifier molecules act as intermediary to bind both water and oil. These types of chemical compounds are of utmost importance to living processes and for the manufacture of cosmetic products.

To create an emulsion, oil, an emulsifier, and water must be mixed in a way that finely disperses the oil in water (or vice versa). Depending on the emulsifier used, two types of emulsions can be created: oil in water (O/W) emulsions or water in oil (W/O) emulsions. The first disperses oil droplets in water and the second disperses water droplets in oil. Note in Figure 19 how sites with affinity to oil on the emulsifier molecules attach themselves to oil droplets in O/W emulsions and how sites with affinity to water on the emulsifier molecule attach themselves to water droplets in W/O emulsions. Most good creams and lotions are O/W emulsions and contain up to 80 percent water. Sometimes it is desirable to have a cream with a little more resistance to water when used as a sunscreen or for environmental and occupational protection. For these types of applications W/O creams are formulated. If you want to know what kind of emulsion your favorite cream or lotion is made of, put some on your finger and let water run over it. If it washes off easily it is an O/W product, if not, it is of the W/O kind.

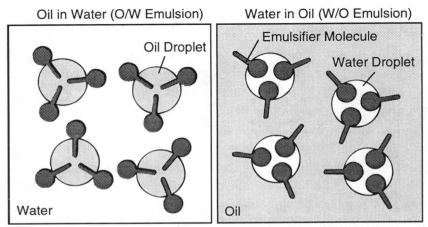

Fig. 19 *Two kinds of emulsion, oil in water and water in oil*

Mono- and diglycerides represent an important class of emulsifiers but they are by no means the only ones. Other natural compounds, like phospholipids, alginates and a large number of synthetic chemicals, perform very similar functions using the same basic principles. Of the 600 most popular emulsifiers used in today's cosmetic products only a small percentage are of natural origin.

Lecithin: A Natural Emulsifier

Lecithin is made up of many different types of phospholipids which are naturally occurring emulsifying agents. Phospholipids are one of the principal components of living cell membranes, where their unique structures are involved both in containing the cell and allowing special protein molecules to selectively transport ions and other substances through the membrane. With the conceptual, technical knowledge of the formation of oils and fats from glycerine and fatty acids, you are now in a position to understand the very similar structure of phosphoglycerides which are also the active and beneficial components of lecithin for skin care. Phosphoglycerides look like triglycerides except that one of the fatty

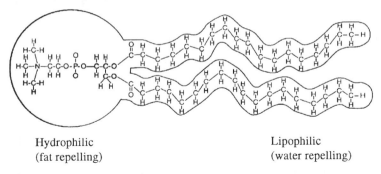

Hydrophilic
(fat repelling)

Lipophilic
(water repelling)

Fig. 20 *Conceptual shape of phospholipid molecule*

acid chains is substituted by a phosphate compound (phosphate ester). The conceptual picture is shown in Figure 20. The phosphor compound increases the water affinity of the glyceride, giving it the unique quality to act as an emulsifier, just like the mono- and diglycerides described in the previous section.

Phospholipids are completely harmless to your body and skin. They are natural emulsifiers that are a component of the very skin cells that cosmetic products are trying to protect and rejuvenate. The most important commercial source of phospholipids is lecithin, a by-product of soybean oil production. Another source for phospholipids used in cosmetics are poultry eggs. The two most important phospholipid compounds in lecithin are phosphatidylcholine (PC) and phosphatidylethanolamine (PE) occurring in concentrations of about 23 percent and 20 percent respectively. The uses of phospholipids in cosmetic products are manifold. They are superior skin restorative agents, moisturizers, and have the ability to penetrate the epidermis and carry substances right to the cell level. They can form cell-like structures called liposomes, which are more fully described in the section on humectants.

Lecithin is seldom used in appreciable amounts in today's cosmetics because of the high cost of the purified compounds and the difficulty in formulating stable products. Phospholipids are amber colored and give the finished product a beige-colored appearance. You will find products containing phospholipids mainly advertised in high priced products and as anti-aging and anti-wrinkle creams and lotions.

Synthetic Emulsifiers

There are very few synthetic emulsifiers that are harmless. Most of the rest have shown a long history of adverse reactions in humans and lack the many benefits of lecithin products. In my survey I found that over 80 percent of emulsifiers used in cosmetic products in the United States today have caused adverse skin reactions in the past. The majority of them may contain toxic contaminants whose long-term systemic effects have not been studied. Emulsifiers are probably the single greatest cause of adverse reactions, and together with perfumes, are the most suspect for causing dermatitis and containing toxic by-products. Below is a brief description of the most commonly used groups of emulsifiers in cosmetic products:

Alkoxylated Alcohols: These compounds are synthesized by reacting an alcohol with ethylene oxide or other alkylene oxides. Ethylene oxide is a potent poison and some of it can be left in the final product after the reaction is completed. Furthermore, 1,4-dioxane, a potent carcinogen, is generated in the process and cannot be completely removed. On product labels they are listed as ingredients ending with - eth (like laureth-n), and ingredient names containing the syllable -oxynol-, PEG (polyethylene glycol), polyethylene, and PPG (polypropylene glycol). Adverse effects on skin caused by products containing alkoxylated alcohols is well documented in the medical literature. Recent analysis of a cross section of cosmetic products confirms the continuing problem with dioxane (see Ref. 179).

Alkoxylated Amides: These emulsifiers are synthesized from fatty acids with primary or secondary alkanolamines. Some of the commonly used alkanolamines are diethanolamine (DEA), monoethanolamine (MEA), triethanolamine (TEA), and monoisopropanolamine (MIPA). On product labels they are listed with the acid name in the front, followed by the syllable "amide," followed by the alkanolamine used in the synthesis. Examples are acetamide MEA, cocamide DEA, and stearamide MEA. All compounds including DEA, MEA, TEA, and MIPA can undergo nitrosation in the skin and body and form nitrosamines which have been determined to form cancer in laboratory animals (see Ref. 150). The FDA has repeatedly expressed concern in the past about the contamination of cosmetic products with nitrosamines.

Alkoxylated Amines: These groups of ingredients appear on product labels with the prefix PEG-n, or poloxamine-n. They suffer from the same contaminations and side effects as those listed under alkoxylated alcohols above.

Alkoxylated Carboxylic (fatty) Acids: These emulsifiers are synthesized from polyethylene glycol (an alcohol) and one of the many fatty acids to form an ester or ether. On the label of cosmetic products they appear as: PEG-n plus name of a fatty acid salt, like PEG-8 Laurate (salt of lauric acid). All chemicals with the designation PEG contain some amount of the toxic chemical 1,4-dioxane (Ref. 150) as a manufacturing by-product. Recent analysis of a cross section of cosmetic products confirms the continuing problem with dioxane.

Fatty Alcohols: Fatty alcohols are higher molecular weight non-volatile alcohols that are used as reactive components for the synthesis of a variety of cosmetic chemicals. By themselves they are used as emollients as well as co-emulsifiers to increase viscosity of cosmetic products. Both of the two most popular fatty alcohols used as co-emulsifiers, cetyl alcohol and cetearyl alcohol, have been shown to cause contact eczema (see Ref. 100, 134).

Glyceryl Esters and Derivatives: Plant oils are natural esters formed by glycerine (an alcohol) and fatty acids and are called triglycerides. When one or two fatty acid chains are chemically removed from the triglyceride a new important class of compounds results that has emulsifying properties. They are call monoglycerides if two fatty acid chains have been removed and diglycerides if only one fatty acid chain is missing. The chemical structure of these molecules has been treated in detail at the beginning of this section. These compounds appear on product labels as Glyceryl followed by the name of the fatty acid for monoglycerides (like glyceryl stearate), and Glyceryl Di- followed by the name of the fatty acid for diglycerides (like glyceryl dioleate). Another class of emulsifiers is synthesized with polyethylene glycol and appears with a PEG-n in front of the ingredient name, followed by the above named nomenclature, like PEG-n glyceryl oleate. Many mono- and diglycerides cause skin irritations and allergies with some listed in Appendix A. In addition, all chemicals with the designation PEG can contain some amount of the toxic chemical 1,4-dioxane (Ref. 150) as a manufacturing by-product.

Phosphorus Compounds: Phosphorus compounds are primarily organic esters of ortho-phosphoric acid. Natural phosphorus compounds, called phospholipids, are very valuable and non-toxic emulsifiers and have been described in detail at the beginning of this section. Of the synthetic phosphorus compounds mostly those containing alkoxylated fatty alcohols or amines are used in cosmetics. On the labels they are listed as phosphorus compounds ending with -eth, like laureth-n and containing the syllable -oxynol-, PEG (propylene glycol), polyethylene, and PPG (polypropylene glycol). Some of the commonly used alkanolamines are diethanolamine (DEA), monoethanolamine (MEA), and monoisopropanolamine (MIPA). All those emulsifiers have the same adverse effects on the skin, and can contain the same toxic compounds as mentioned under alkoxylated alcohols and amides.

Sorbitan Derivatives: Sorbitol is a naturally occurring organic sugar-like compound. In synthetic form it is used as raw material for a number of cosmetic and food products. Sorbic alcohols react with fatty acids to form esters that are excellent emulsifiers. They are used in food products as well as in cosmetic preparations. These emulsifiers appear on product labels as Sorbitan followed by the name of the fatty acid if one fatty acid is attached (like sorbitan stearate), and Sorbitan Di- followed by the name of the fatty acid if two fatty acids are attached (like sorbitan dioleate). Another group of sorbitan emulsifiers is synthesized with polyethylene glycol and appears with the prefix PEG on product labels. As mentioned above, all chemicals with the designation PEG can contain some amount of the toxic chemical 1,4-dioxane as a manufacturing by-product.

Soaps and Shampoos

Pure water, used by itself, is our most important cleansing substance. It gently removes all emulsified substances from the skin and hair without damage to the natural protective mantle of the skin. It also removes all soluble environmental pollutants from your skin like nitrogen and sulfur compounds, metal salts, and most of the occupational chemicals to which you may be exposed. Soaps are needed to remove greasy substances that cannot be dissolved by water.

Recipes for soaps appear on cuneiform clay tablets of the Sumerians more than 6,000 years ago and on Egyptian murals and papyri dating from about 2,000 B.C. Soaps were manufactured from plant ashes containing alkali and from animal or plant fats containing triglycerides of various fatty acids. Soap was considered a luxury article and those free citizens of Rome who could afford a visit to a Roman bath received a piece of soap when paying their entry fees. According to Pliny, soaps were made during the period of the Roman Empire by boiling goat tallow with wood ashes.

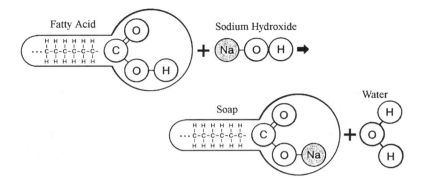

Fig. 21 *Making soap from fatty acids*

The art of soap making was further developed during the Middle Ages in Europe, mainly in France, Italy, and Spain. The soaps from Venice became world famous and the "Savon de Marseille" became a sought-after article because of its fine quality. They were mostly made from tallow, which is still used today for soap production. These early soaps were not too skin-friendly but certainly cleaned well. They had a big advantage over today's synthetic cleaning substances: they were fully biodegradable and did not pollute rivers and lakes.

To form soap, a natural fat must be completely broken down into its molecular components, which are glycerine and fatty acids. This is accomplished by heating fats in an alkali solution. During this process the fatty acid reacts with the metal ion in the heated alkaline solution to form a fatty acid salt which is called soap, with glycerine being freed in the process. A conceptual picture of this process, called saponification, and the shape of a soap molecule is shown in Figure 21.

How Soaps Work

As shown previously, fatty acid molecules consist of a head with small affinity to water and a tail with a large affinity to oil. In the saponification process the oil-loving or lipophilic tail stays intact while the addition of a positively charged metal ion makes the head strongly water loving or hydrophilic. This gives the soap molecule very similar properties to those of the emulsifiers discussed in the previous section. In the washing process, the lipophilic tail attaches itself to oils and fats on the skin surface and disperses them into the surrounding water (see Figure 22). In the process of cleansing, soaps destroy the natural protective mantle of the skin (which can take several hours to re-establish itself). Harsh soaps and detergents can also leach out the phospholipid content of the epidermis and leave a damaged skin barrier that can be more easily penetrated by chemicals and bacteria.

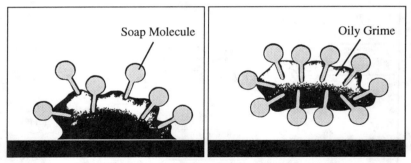

Fig. 22 *How soap molecules disperse oily grime*

Synthetic Soaps (Surfactants)

Modern synthetic surfactants (liquid soaps) share the same fundamental molecular structure with conventional soaps and emulsifying agents: a lipophilic fatty acid tail and a hydrophilic head composed of various organic and non-organic compounds (see Figure 23). Similar to phospholipids, surfactant molecules are able to form membrane-like structures (bubbles). This attribute, and their ability to decrease surface tensions in liquids, is manifest by their foaming action or formation of soap bubbles as shown in Figure 24. For these reason, soaps and emulsifying agents are called surface active agents, or surfactants. There are some

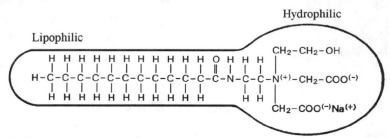

Fig. 23 *Conceptual shape of surefactant molecule (glycine derivative)*

surfactants that occur naturally in plants. Some of them, like soapwort (saponaria officinalis), served our ancestors as washes and for medicinal purposes. They consist of betaines and saponins and have served as models for the synthesis of modern surfactants and detergents.

Using the large number of available compounds, modern chemistry has created an enormous number of different surfactants that are responsible for the creation of a large and profitable industry. At first, little thought was given to skin compatibility and biodegradability of these synthetic products. The detergent industry eventually created huge environmental problems in the 1960s by infesting rivers and lakes and killing aquatic life. This continued until governmental regulations in most countries forbade the use of some of

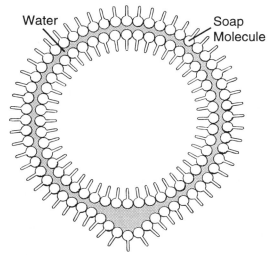

Water Soap Molecule

Fig. 24 *Formation of bubbles by detergents*

the most damaging variety of surfactants. The first surfactants marketed for skin and hair care had great cleansing powers but were so brutal to the skin that the medical profession soon sounded the alarm. Those that used them to shower and bathe every day soon developed eczema and dermatitis. Since industry did not bother to conduct sufficient research on the long-term effect of surfactants on the human skin, this situation resulted in the largest unauthorized chemical compatibility test on an unsuspecting population in history. The most damaging products were taken off the market, but many of the questionable compounds remain. This test is still in process today with thousands of people suffering from redness due to dermatitis when using liquid soaps, hair shampoos, bath preparations, and dish washing detergents.

My survey shows that more than 50 percent of all the surfactants listed on cosmetic labels in the U.S. have medical evidence of causing adverse effects on the human skin. They are identified in Appendix A. I recommend that you stop using products that list such ingredients even if you have not developed visible adverse reactions. Studies have shown that many of the harsh surfactants deplete natural fats and phospholipids from the epidermis, weakening the natural barrier and allowing toxic substances and bacteria to invade the skin. Many surfactants also contain toxic contaminants that are created during the manufacturing process.

Properties of Synthetic Surfactants

Alkanoamides: These surfactants (detergents) are synthesized from fatty acids with primary or secondary alkanolamines. Some of the commonly used alkanolamines are diethanolamine (DEA), monoethanolamine (MEA), and monoisopropanolamine (MIPA). All compounds including DEA, MEA, and MIPA can undergo nitrosation in the skin and body and form nitrosamines which have been determined to form cancer in laboratory animals (see Appendix A.) –The FDA has repeatedly expressed concern about the contamination of cosmetic products with nitrosamines in the past. They are used in cosmetics in shampoos as detergents and foam boosters and to enhance viscosity.

Alkoxylated Alcohols: Alkoxylated alcohols are ethers formed from alcohols and alkylene oxides (ethylene or propylene oxide). During the process 1,4-dioxane, a potent carcinogen, is generated that and it cannot be completely removed. On the label they are listed as ingredients ending with -eth, like laureth-n, ingredient names containing the syllable -oxynol-, PEG (polyethylene glycol), polyethylene, and PPG (polypropylene glycol). There are many references in the medical literature about adverse effects on skin caused by products containing alkoxylated alcohols. Recent analysis of a cross section of cosmetic products confirms the continuing problem with dioxane (see Appendix A). Alkoxylated alcohols form a large number of different chemicals that are widely used in cosmetics as detergents, solubilizers, and conditioners.

Alkoxylated Amides: These surfactants are synthesized from fatty acids with primary or secondary alkanolamines. Some of the commonly used alkanolamines are diethanolamine (DEA), monoethanolamine (MEA), triethanolamine (TEA), and monoisopropanolamine (MIPA). On product labels they are listed with the acid name first, followed by the syllable -amide- , followed by the alkanolamine used in the synthesis. Examples are acetamide MEA; cocamide DEA, or stearamide MEA. All compounds including DEA, MEA, TEA and MIPA can undergo nitrosation in the skin and body and form nitrosamines which have been determined to form cancer in laboratory animals (see Appendix A). The FDA has repeatedly expressed concern about the contamination of cosmetic products with nitrosamines in the past (Ref. 150).

Alkylamido Alkylamines: Commercially available alkylamido alkylamines are complex mixtures of chemically related surfactants. They are amphoteric in nature (see glossary) and leave the hair conditioned after shampooing. You can spot them on the ingredient label easily because they contain the syllable -ampho-, like sodium lauramphoacetate. They are mild and substantive and are frequently used as baby shampoos.

Alkyl Polyglucosides: Although described first over hundred years ago in the chemical literature, this class of surfactants is only recently being produced commercially. The initial raw materials are glucose (a sugar) and fatty acids with various carbon chain lengths. The resulting compounds are very mild surfactants with good skin and hair compatibility. They are fully biodegradable and no adverse effects have been identified so far.

Alkyl Ether Sulfates: These surfactants are synthesized from alkoxylated alcohols and sulfuric acid. They have similar properties as listed under alkoxylated alcohols and may contain dioxane and/or nitroso compounds. They are excellent cleansers and have good foaming properties.

Alkyl-Substituted Amino Acids: This type of surfactants, containing amino acids (like glycine), are is more fully treated in the text under "Gentle Cleansing Ingredients." They can be spotted on the ingredients label by looking for names of amino acids, like glycine or glycinate. They are used in all types of cleansing products where mildness and compatibility with active ingredients are required.

Alkyl Sulfates: Alkyl sulfates and alkyl ether sulfates are related compounds and are synthesized from fatty alcohols and/or alkoxylated alcohols, sulfuric acid and a base, like sodium hydroxide. A combination of all three components are usually listed on the ingredient label, always containing the syllable -sulfate-, like sodium lauryl sulfate. Those products that use organic bases for the synthesis, like DEA, MEA, and TEA, may undergo nitrosation and form cancerous nitrosamines. Alkyl sulfates and alkyl ether sulfates are widely used in shampoos and other cleansing applications. They have good cleansing and foaming properties but at the same time can cause skin irritations in a large sector of users (see Appendix A).

Betaines: Betaines are complicated organic detergents that occur naturally in sugar beets and other plants. The synthesized versions of betaines are amphoteric compounds and are widely used in the cosmetic industry as mild detergents and foaming agents, and as skin and hair conditioners. There are few reports in the literature about adverse effects of betaines.

Protein Derivatives: Especially mild detergents can be made from various hydrolyzed animal proteins (like elastin and collagen) and plant proteins that are joined with fatty acids and neutralized with organic or inorganic bases. Their names on ingredient labels consist of the names of the base, fatty acid, and the words "hydrolyzed protein," like potassium-coco-hydrolyzed animal protein. They form a group of mild surfactants except that those compounds with prefix TEA (triethanol amine) and MEA (monoethanolamine) may form nitrosamines, a known cancer producing agent.

Soaps: Soaps were the first surface active agents and their manufacture and effectiveness is explained in the beginning of this section. They are metal salts of fatty acids and are, as a rule, very effective and aggressive cleansers. They are still widely used as cosmetic cleansers with little side effects.

Gentle Cleansing Substances

Modern chemistry has changed our everyday life to a considerable degree. Although it has developed some toxic substances, it has also surrounded us with many conveniences like plastics, synthetic fibers, dyes, motor fuel, medicines, and, believe it or not, gentle washing substances. Chemists have been hard at work during the last decade and have succeeded in partly using natural substances to synthesize surfactants. One of these products is made from collagen, an essential part of human and animal skin. Although the building blocks of basic protein molecules are very small (see Chapter 3 on skin care), collagen contains thousands of basic protein building blocks chained together in what is called a fibrous protein. The

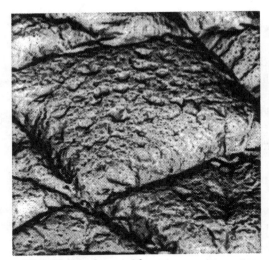

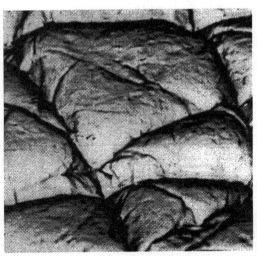

Fig. 25 *Washtest without sucrose cocoate (GRILLO)*

Fig. 26 *Washtest with 2% sucrose cocoate (GRILLO)*

collagen protein chains are hydrophilic and are responsible for retaining most of the water in the human skin. Even when broken into smaller pieces (hydrolyzed) and chemically joined to natural fatty acids, they retain their hydrophilic character and when bound to the lipophilic fatty acid can form a very gentle washing substance. Mild surfactants can also be made using simple amino acids that are basic building blocks for proteins like glycine, arginine, or glutamic acid. Instead of a long protein chain (as in the previous example), a single amino acid provides the hydrophilic part when bonded to a fatty acid chain. These types of surfactants are especially mild.

Chemists have recently succeeded in creating surfactants whose attributes consumers and environmentalists have been dreaming of for years. They are completely non-toxic for plants, animals and man, are completely biodegradable, and can be safely discharged into the environment. These products are made from glucose (sugar) and fatty acids. They are designated on labels as sucrose and polyglucose derivatives with the name of a fatty acid added (like sucrose cocoate). A quantity of only two percent added to detergents decreases the irritation factor of products from five- to six-fold. Figures 25 and 26 compare greatly enlarged parts of skin surfaces following a wash test. The skin surface in Figure 25 has been washed repeatedly with one of the most popular and inexpensive surfactants on the market today, sodium lauryl ether sulfate. Figure 26 represents a skin surface washed with a surfactant containing two percent sucrose cocoate. The skin surface cleaned with sodium lauryl ether sulfate has part of the phospholipids content of the epidermis removed so that it appears pitted and rough. The skin treated with the surfactant containing sucrose cocoate is smooth and the phospholipid barrier seems to be completely intact. A small amount of this substance added to your dish washing liquid would permanently eliminate skin irritation from your hands. Polyglucosides have similar properties and can be used as a super mild primary surfactants in cosmetic preparations.

I highly recommend products made of these and similar mild surfactants. As with emulsifying agents, these substances are more expensive and are harder to work with for the cosmetic formulator. Below is a brief description of the most commonly used groups of synthetic surfactants in cosmetic products.

Humectants

The main purpose of any cream or lotion is to keep the skin moist and elastic and prevent the upper skin layer from drying out. Many conventional moisturizing creams and lotions form an occlusive film on the skin to prevent water loss. This prevention of water loss can cause an increase in hydration of the epidermal layer or unwanted swelling of the skin tissue. This is frequently observed when a thick layer of fatty night cream is left on the face until morning causing your facial tissues to swell. Some moisturizing agents are strongly hygroscopic (like glycerine). They attract water from the surrounding air as well as from the tissues. They will keep the surface moist as long as there is sufficient moisture in the air. In a dry climate they defeat their purpose as skin moisturizers because they are drying out the skin underneath to satisfy their hunger for water.

Phospholipids

There are several outstanding natural moisturizers that can be used with great confidence since they are completely non-toxic and non-irritating. In a recent study titled Phospholipids as Moisturizing Agents by Alec D. Keith and Wallace Snipes (edited by Phillip Frost), several important attributes of topically applied phosphatidylcholine (PC) and phosphatidylethanolamine (PE) were discussed. [5] They observed that the horny layer or epidermis is composed of about 20 layers of keratinized cells that still have a significant phospholipid content. Through environmental influences, like abrasion and exposure to detergents and solvents, the cells of the outer level of skin lose a larger than normal amount of phospholipids to the environment which can no longer be replaced by a normal cell repair process (since these cells no longer metabolize). This loss weakens the barrier properties of the horny layer and makes it appear pitted under the microscope and rough to the feel. This study showed some remarkable features of these keratinized cells. It determined that membrane phospholipids of the outer skin can be restored by topical treatment with plant

---

[5]   Frost, Phillip, M.D., Horwitz, Steven N., *Principles of cosmetics for the dermatologist*, The C.V. Mosby Company, 1982.

phospholipids. The study also highlighted the importance of the phospholipid membrane in the horny layer to protect the skin from outside substances like bacteria and harmful chemicals.

The study also showed that phospholipids, being a natural component of the membrane system, are hygroscopic (attract water from the surrounding air) and hold water in place where an increased level of hydration is needed. In this manner phospholipids increase the hydration level of the skin without modifying the water loss rate of the skin. Another beneficial property of phospholipids depends on their unsaturated fatty acid content. Phosphatidylcholine (PC), one of the components of lecithin from vegetable sources, contains a high percentage of unsaturated fatty acid chains (70% linoleic acid and 6% linolenic acid). They are referred to in Europe as Vitamin F and have been found essential for fat metabolism and for the release of fat from fatty tissues. In a recent German study it was concluded that linoleic acid is one of the most valuable ingredients in cosmetics. [6] The study found that a shortage of linoleic acid increases acne formation, and that the water loss from skin is inversely proportional to the linoleic acid content of the skin. Another compound that has been shown to be a deep moisturizer and that contains the single unsaturated fatty acid, linoleic acid, is vitamin E linoleate. Therefore, unsaturated fatty acid compounds should be a part of every serious moisturizing skin care product.

Liposomes

A most important and interesting attributes of phospholipids are their ability to form special microscopic molecular structures called liposomes. With our recently acquired conceptual background of molecular shapes and chemistry, we are now able to visualize one of the secrets of life and the formation and attributes of liposomes. As previously mentioned, the shape of a phospholipid molecule consists of a water-loving head and two oil-loving tails. When placing a large number of these molecules into a limited space they will arrange themselves spontaneously to match their heads together and also their tails. Figure 27 shows the arrangement of a section of a living cell membrane which consists largely of phospholipids. As you can see, the phospholipid molecules have arranged themselves to form a membrane so that oil droplets cannot penetrate the cell membrane because they would be repelled by the wall of hydrophilic heads. In like manner, no water can penetrate the membrane because the lipophilic tails inside will not allow passage. The only access through the membrane is by special protein molecules that are programmed to let only certain chemicals pass in and out of the cell

---

[6] Lautenschlager, H. Md., Roedinger J. Md, Ghyczy, M. Md., The Use of Liposomes from Soybean Phospholipids in Cosmetics, *SÖFW*, issue 14/88, p. 531-534.

Cell Membrane

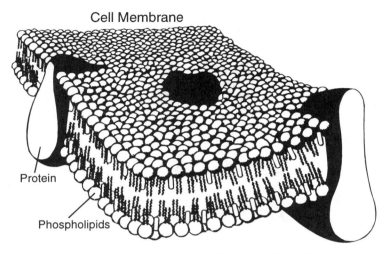

Protein

Phospholipids

Fig. 27 *Phospholipids forming human cell membrane*

Plant phospholipids are all very similar in structure and composition. Under certain physical conditions they will spontaneously form microscopic spheres whose walls are very similar in construction to the actual cell membrane shown in Figure 28. The size of these spheres are very small — in the order of a nanometer. As illustrated, the spheres are hollow inside and enclose some of the liquid material in which they were formed (inclusion).Because of the small size of the phospholipid molecule and microspheres, they can pass through the epidermis and act as a carrier for the enclosed substances. It is postulated that when they reach the outside of a living cell membrane in the dermis they may become accepted as part of the membrane, being of the same composition. This process is as shown in Figure 29.

Thus, they are able to carry with them any enclosed substances into the dermis and to the individual cells.

This attribute of phospholipids and the carrier mechanism for delivering active ingredients directly to the cell level has extensive implications for cosmetics. By themselves they are absolutely non-toxic and cause no skin irritations, not even around the eyes. Their danger lies in their ability to carry toxic or contaminated substances into the cells. The development of liposome technology offers the potential for many cosmetic products. However, the cosmetic developer has to deal

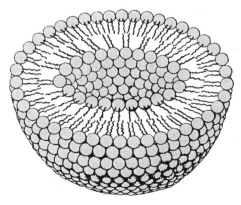

Fig. 28 *Liposome structure formed by phospholipids*

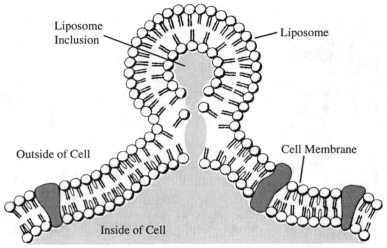

Fig. 29 *Acceptance of liposomes into living cells*

very carefully with the selection of raw materials and the question of the biological fate of the preparation. The microspheres themselves are constantly undergoing changes due to thermal activity during preparation and storage. As a result, each ingredient of the preparation can end up inside the microspheres over time. More than 80 percent of the cosmetic products on the market contain toxic substances that if used in liposome products will eventually become part of the inclusion inside liposomes that, in turn, will get inside your skin cells. Therefore, beware of products with liposomes that also contain substances that cause adverse effects. As an example, preservatives fall into this hazardous category since they are all cellular toxins.

It has not been decided by the FDA whether liposome products with inclusions should be considered as medicine and put under the scrutiny of medical doctors with the advantage of documenting and tracking long-term adverse effects. According to the Cosmetic Handbook, published by the Food and Drug Administration, "Products that are cosmetics but are also intended to treat or prevent disease, or affect the structure or functions of the human body, are considered also drugs and must comply with both the drug and cosmetic provisions of the law." [7] Some combinations of liposomes and active substances certainly qualify for this category. The cosmetic industry has no intention of waiting for a decision before cashing in on the remarkable properties of liposomes.

---

[7]   U.S. Department of Health and Human Services, *Cosmetic Handbook*, U.S. Government Printing Office.

Proteins

Topically applied extracts of hydrolyzed proteins have enjoyed a great popularity in the past as humectants. Natural animal proteins consist of giant chains of amino acids, the basic building blocks of life. They contain a large number of different amino acids joined chemically by a peptide bond. The most important proteins used in cosmetics are collagen, elastin, and keratin. Collagen is a tough and fibrous protein and is the most common protein

Table 2 Amino Acid Content in Percent of Typical Protein Hydrolysates

Amino Acid	Collagen	Keratin	Elastin	Wheat Protein
Alanine	9.7	4.1	16.7	2.7
Arginine	7.9	9.5	1.8	3.3
Aspartic acid	5.0	8.3	2.5	3.2
Glutamic acid	9.5	15.5	4.3	40.2
Glycine	25.9	5.2	20.9	3.3
Histidin	0.5	0.2	0.3	2.4
Hydroxyproline	10.5	-	2.6	-
Leucine/Isoleucine	4.5	11.7	10.7	11.8
Lysine	3.7	2.7	1.5	1.6
Methionine	-	-	0.1	1.6
Phenylalanine	2.0	3.2	6.3	5.7
Proline	13.0	6.4	14.5	14.3
Serine	3.3	8.5	1.7	5.2
Threonine	1.6	6.2	1.4	2.8
Tyrosine	0.6	3.8	1.5	3.8
Valine	2.1	4.9	12.0	4.7
Cystine/Cysteic acid	-	9.9	-	2.2
Desmosine	-	-	0.7	-
Isodesmosine	-	-	0.3	-

in animals. Elastin forms elastic and stretchable connecting tissues throughout the animal body. Keratin is the main constituent of hair, nails and the outer layer of the skin. It is resistant to a wide range of chemicals and physical abrasion. In their natural form most of the proteins are unsuitable for use in cosmetic products. They must be converted into soluble hydrolysates, or in other words, broken into smaller parts by treatment with acids or enzymes. Depending on the final size of the resulting molecules, protein hydrolysates form thick gels with waters (gelatin) that are not suitable for use in cosmetic products, or viscous solutions that are used as skin conditioning agents and for manufacturing surfactants. The approximate amino acid content for soluble proteins, including that for wheat protein, are given in Table 2. Both plant and animal proteins have excellent skin compatibility and deposit a protective film on the skin or hair. This film has smoothing and moisturizing effect and reduces the potential for irritation due to external (and product based) agents. Some cosmetic companies want to make you believe that special animal proteins can be used by your skin to rejuvenate and replace aging cells. However, a simple calculation of the size of collagen or elastin molecules, even when broken down (hydrolyzed), show that they are orders of magnitude too large to pass through the tightly packed horny layer of the skin. Even if you could get them into the dermal layer, by injection for instance, they would be immediately rejected and attacked by the body's immune system.

A similar case can be made for cambium, which are special cells found in living plant tissues that are responsible for the new growth in plants above and below ground. These cells do not age and are active in some plants for over a thousand years. The connection is obvious, treat your skin with those immortal cells and forget about aging. Again, this is absolute nonsense. The argument against their use is similar to the one made against animal proteins. They are much too large to penetrate the horny layer of the skin to get into the lower skin layers. Even if they could, they would immediately be attacked by the body's immune system.

Synthetic Humectants

My study found that a large percentage of synthetic moisturizers listed on cosmetic product labels in the U.S. are causing adverse reactions in some section of the population. The following is a description of groups of the most common synthetic humectants you will find in skin creams and lotions and some hair conditioners:

Alcohols and Polyols: Alcohols form a large number of chemical compounds, many of which have familiar names, like ethanol (grain alcohol), propanol (propyl alcohol), glycol, propanetriol (glycerine). While grain alcohol is a harsh solvent, higher alcohols and polyols are oily to solid substances, some of which are used as humectants. Propylene glycol is probably the most common humectant found in skin creams and lotions because it is antibacterial, a good solvent for various plant materials, and a stabilizer for emulsions.

Unfortunately, it also causes irritation and contact dermatitis in many users. Several additional alcohols used as humectants, including glycol, glycerol (glycerine), also cause contact dermatitis (Ref. 90).

Alkoxylated Alcohols: Alkoxylated alcohols have been described in the emulsifier section of this chapter. Several compounds in this category are used as humectants as well and are designated on the labels of cosmetic products as glycereth, -gluceth-n, and PEG-n. As was mentioned before, 1,4-dioxane, a potent carcinogen, is generated in the synthesis and cannot be completely removed. Adverse effects on skin caused by products containing alkoxylated alcohols is well documented in the medical literature. Recent analysis of a cross section of cosmetic products confirms the continuing problem with dioxane (see Appendix A).

Amides and Amines: Humectants in this category include acetamide-MEA, compounds starting with the syllable TEA (triethanolamine), and glucamine. As was pointed out in the emulsifier section, all compounds including MEA, TEA, and MIPA can undergo nitrosation in the skin and body. The FDA has repeatedly expressed concern about the contamination of cosmetic products with cancer-causing nitrosamines in the past.

Preservatives

Microorganisms are tiny single-celled living organisms too small to be seen by the naked eye. They can be found everywhere on the surface of the earth, in the air, and especially on your skin. A square inch of skin can be the habitat of 100,000 or more of these organisms. Most of them are quite harmless to the healthy individual. They perform many useful functions, such as aiding with the digestion of food in our intestines. A relative minority of them are disease causing (pathogenic) microorganisms and must be carefully guarded against. Among them are bacteria (which cause diphtheria, food poisoning, pneumonia, and typhoid), viruses (which cause many infections including AIDS, the common cold, influenza, and measles), protozoa (which is an organism that causes amebic dysentery, giardiasis, and malaria), fungi (which cause disorders such as ringworm and thrush), and rickettsiae (which is the causative agent for typhus and Rocky Mountain spotted fever) and more.

Microorganisms would multiply freely in cosmetic products unless special substances, called preservatives, were added to inhibit their growth. The Food and Drug Administration guidelines do not require cosmetic products to be sterile or free from living microorganisms, but they do require that products not be contaminated with pathogenic (disease causing) organisms. No permissible concentration of pathogenic or non-pathogenic organisms is mentioned, except that it must be low and must remain in this condition when used by the consumer. In other words, the concentration of preservatives in the product must be sufficiently high to inhibit the growth of microorganisms during its use by the consumer.

A cream or lotion initially free from microorganism and without added preservatives would last only eight to fourteen days before spoiling after opening. Even if refrigerated, its useful life to the consumer would be only about four weeks. Products containing no preservatives must be filled in a bacteria-free environment and would have an expiration date, like milk and other perishable products in the supermarkets, and would have to be checked checked to remove expired products. Cosmetic manufacturers cannot perform this service; for this reason they add enough preservatives to their products to ensure a shelf life of two to three years. This allows them to produce large batches of products and not worry about spoilage. As a result, the list of medical publications about adverse reactions due to preservatives in cosmetics is long.

Table 3 Cosmetic Preservatives with Adverse Reactions

benzylparaben	bronopol
butylated hydroxytoluene (BHT)	butylated hydroxyanisole(BHA)
butylparaben	chloromethylisothiazolinone
dibromocyanobutane	diazolidinyl urea
dichlorophen	dichlorobenzyl alcohol
DMD hydantoin	dimethyl hydroxymethyl pyrazole
ethylparaben	ethyl-p-hydroxybenzoate
isothiazolinone	imidazolidinyl urea
methylparaben	methenammonium chloride
methyldibromo glutaronitrile	methylchloroisothiazolinone
phenoxyethanol	methylisothiazolinone
propylparaben	propyl benzoate
sodium sulphosuccinate	sodium hydroxymethylglycinate
thiomersal	

The industry and FDA consider the use of preservatives an acceptable risk because the alternative of not using them is worse and more dangerous. Table 3 is a summary, extracted from Appendix A, that lists almost all preservatives on the market today that have caused harmful skin reaction in consumers of cosmetic products. You will probably find the preservative listed on your skin and hair care products among them.

The majority of manufacturers preserve their products with a combination of parabens and diazolidinyl urea because they are relatively safe. Nevertheless, all preservatives are cellular toxins and as such need to be handled carefully. Figure 30 shows the warning label on all commercial paraben containers that are shipped to cosmetic manufactures.

WARNING:	This is a highly concentrated paraben solution and therefore causes severe eyeburns and skin irritation. In cases of contact immediately flush with plenty of water for at least 15 minutes. For eye contact seek medical attention.
CAUTION:	For manufacturing use only. The user assumed all risks in handling. The supplier makes no warranty of any kind, expressed or implied, concerning its use.

Fig. 30 *Warning label on industrial paraben container*

My survey shows that over 80 percent of all preservatives listed on product labels in the U.S. have caused allergic skin reactions and dermatitis. Some are carcinogenic and others are believed to cause possible systemic reactions even though they have not been studied. There are at least two ways to minimize the adverse effect due to preservatives. The first is to produce products with a limited shelf life and with a stated expiration date. This would allow the use of natural preservatives (such as essential oils) with fewer side effects. The second is to produce products without preservatives that would require special preparation and filling and refrigeration once opened. Neither of the above alternatives is likely to be adopted by large cosmetic companies because of the logistic nightmare it would create for suppliers. Eventually some smaller companies may adopt the first approach to give the consumer a choice of better protection.

Natural Preservatives

Essential oils are natural substances that are powerful preservatives and that are not extensively used to preserve cosmetic products. They are derived from flowers, leaves, grasses, and woody plants. The first indications of their antiseptic properties were uncovered during the cholera epidemics of the nineteenth century in France when tens of thousands of men, women, and children perished. During this time it was observed that workers in perfume factories were almost completely immune to this disease. Today we know that most essential oils and absolutes used in perfumes are powerful antiseptics that kill most of the harmful bacteria and fungi without harming the human system. The addition of as little as one drop of sweet orange oil to two ounces of cream will kill all bacteria and fungi in the preparation. Essential oils have also been shown to be effective in killing the virus that causes Herpes and assist in healing the affected skin.

Table 4 Effectiveness of Essential Oils in killing Bacteria

Essential oil	Minimum Amount in %	Essential oil	Minimum Amount in %
Thyme	0.070	Rosemary	0.430
Origanum	0.100	Cumin	0.450
Sweet Orange	0.120	Neroli	0.475
Lemongrass	0.160	Birch	0.480
Chinese Cinnamon	0.170	Lavender	0.500
Rose	0.180	Melissa Balm	0.520
Clove	0.200	Ylang Ylang	0.560
Eucalyptus	0.225	Juniper	0.600
Peppermint	0.250	Sweet Fennel	0.640
Rose geranium	0.250	Garlic	0.650
Meadowsweet	0.330	Lemon	0.700
Chinese anise	0.370	Cajeput	0.720
Orris	0.380	Sassafras	0.750
Cinnamon	0.400	Heliotrope	0.800
Wild Thyme	0.400	Fir, Pine	0.860
Anise	0.420	Parsley	0.880
Mustard	0.420	Violet	0.900

Recent studies performed in France determined the potency of essential oils as antiseptics. [8] Increasing amounts of different essential oils were added to meat stock cultured

---

[8]   Valnet, Jean, [Treatment of Illnesses with Plant Oils] *Treatment des Maladies par les essences des Plantes*, Maloine S.A., Editeur, Paris, 1986.

in raw sewage to determine the quantity needed to kill all microorganisms. Table 4 lists the amount of essential oil in percent that must be added to raw sewage to kill all microbes. As can be seen from the table, one part of origanum oil renders 1,000 parts of raw sewage free of all living organisms.

Some of the reasons why essential oils are not more frequently used as preservatives are price (which averages $50 per pound wholesale), odor, and the fact that essential oils are volatile and evaporate from the preparation when left uncovered. Some essential oils also cause reddening of the skin and dermatitis. Products with a larger content of essential oils, as found in aromatherapeutic preparations (foam baths, soaps, bath oils, and massage oils), do not need the addition of harmful synthetic preservatives because of the antiseptic properties of essential oils.

Antioxidants

Atmospheric oxygen plays a major role in spoiling the natural oils used in creams and lotions. Especially vulnerable are compounds that contain polyunsaturated fatty acid chains. These are especially valuable for human nutrition and skin care (see section on emollients and humectants). When broken down by oxygen, fatty acids get the characteristic rancid smell and can form compounds that are called fatty acid peroxides. They are also called free radicals and are highly reactive particles that, if left unchecked, will go on a destructive rampage inside your skin and body and damage and destroy cells. This damage is irreversible and accelerates the aging process of the body and skin. There is accumulating evidence that link free radicals with the formation of cancer, senility, atherosclerosis, and hypertension.

Fortunately, nature has provided its own remedy to slow down this process. There is much evidence that saturated and polyunsaturated fats will not enter into nearly as many destructive free radical reactions if an adequate amount of vitamin E is present. Vitamin E is nature's own antioxidant and free radical scavenger that acts to block the oxidation that can turn lipids into harmful peroxides. Most natural oils containing polyunsaturated chains also contain some vitamin E. However, the manufacturing process and excessive heating of oils removes this natural antioxidant. Carotene and Vitamin A have a similar effect as has Vitamin C in aqueous solutions. Among synthetic antioxidants you will find gallic acid derivatives (propyl gallate), butylated hydroxytoluene (BHT), and butylated hydroxyanisole (BHA) all of which have caused adverse reactions in the past. Other substances that are used to slow down oxidation are chelating compounds. They remove heavy metal traces that can act as catalysts in the formation of free radicals.

Since adverse effects caused by preservatives will be with us for some time to come, it may be necessary to know which of the preservatives can best be tolerated by individuals. Those who suspect that they are sensitive to a particular preservative or antioxidant should perform a patch test. Patch testing is done by placing small amounts of the different preservatives in question on different areas of the inner forearm or other convenient place.

After twelve to twenty-four hours, the skin is examined for adverse effects that can manifest itself in redness (erythema) or a swelling tumor, or in no reaction at all. This method, of course, can be applied to any doubtful ingredient in cosmetic products. It is routinely done by dermatologists and can be easily done in your home (see chapter on Skin Care).

Sunscreens

As the origin of light, the sun is of great importance to life on earth. Life as we know it would be impossible without light. Therefore, it is no wonder that throughout history the Sun God frequently ranked as the supreme mythological God of most cultures. In some cultures, a sunburn was considered punishment by the Gods. Today, a different kind of sun worshipper flocks to the Southern shores in search of the perfect Florida or California tan. These sun seekers don't always realize that they are endangering their health to the most common form of cancer - skin cancer - and exposing themselves to an increased risk of premature aging of their skin. Almost half a million new cases of skin cancer every year are attributed to solar radiation.

Why is sunlight so dangerous? The sun emits an almost continuous spectrum of electromagnetic radiation that ranges from long wavelength radio waves to the visible part of light and beyond to the short wavelength ultraviolet and high energy x-rays. The energy of these waves is inversely proportional to their wave length. In other words, the shorter the wave length the greater the energy of that part of the solar spectrum. For any reasonable exposure, the human skin is not greatly affected by solar radiation with wave lengths up to about 400 nanometers, or the starting wavelength of near ultraviolet (UV-A) rays. UV-A rays are responsible for the tanning of light-skinned people. However, any light of shorter wave length like far ultraviolet rays (UV-B and UV-C) and beyond, poses a greater danger to the human skin. Fortunately, the very high energy rays of the sun are filtered out by our atmosphere, especially the ozone layer, which passes only rays up to and including UV-B rays. As long as the ozone layer remains intact, the UV-B radiation is the highest energy radiation for which we need protection. It is important, therefore, to protect the ozone layer because it filters out much of the dangerous radiation and protects life on earth.

How does ultraviolet light damage the skin? When solar radiation impinges on the skin it penetrates to varying depths. A wide variety of reactions occur in the uppermost layer of the skin as a result of absorbed UV radiation. Penetration of UV radiation initiates biochemical processes in the skin. The most visible effect is pigmentation, or formation of melanin to protect the skin from further damage. The UV rays do not only initiate biochemical reactions in your skin but are also able to alter a variety of cosmetic chemicals that penetrate your skin. UV radiation can transform otherwise harmless chemicals into toxic substances and cause a variety of adverse reactions. A few of these chemicals, called phototoxins, are listed in Table 5.

Other reactions include damage to the DNA/RNA enzyme repair systems, and cause damage to the collagen and keratin in the connective tissues. This process is called solar or senile elastosis. The skin loses its elasticity because sunburn damages the collagen fibers in the upper part of the skin. These lesions often take the form of horny, calloused, wart-like growths called keratosis. The resulting dry and leathery skin may be enough damage, but keratotic lesions are frequent forerunners of skin cancer. As an example of how solar exposure affects different races, dermatologists point out that it is difficult to determine the age of most dark-skinned people by the texture of their skin. Since their skin is far better protected by a higher content of pigment, it does not suffer the same photo-aging or cancer-causing effect that sunlight has on people with light skin.

Table 5 Phototoxic Cosmetic Chemicals

Phototoxic Cosmetic Chemicals	Reference to Adverse Reaction
2-ethoxyethyl-p-methoxy cinnamate (Cinoxate)	causing photosensitivity, Ref(152, 25.64)
3-carbethoxypsoralen	phototoxin; reacts with UV radiation to yield genotoxin, Ref(19)
4,5,8-trimethylpsoralen	phototoxin; reacts with UV radiation to yield genotoxin, Ref(19)
5-methoxypsoralen	phototoxin; reacts with UV radiation to yield genotoxin, Ref(19)
7-methylpyrido[3,4-c]psoralen	phototoxin; reacts with UV radiation to yield genotoxin, Ref(19)
8-methoxypsoralen (methoxsalen)	phototoxin; reacts with UV radiation to yield genotoxin, Ref(19)
8-methoxypsoralen (methoxsalen)	causing photosensitivity, Ref(152, 25.64)
Cinoxate (2-ethoxyethyl-p-methoxy cinnamate)	causing photosensitivity, Ref(152, 25,64)
cornflower extract	causing allergy and photosensitivity , Ref(120)
cornflower distillate	causing allergy and photosensitivity , Ref(120)

Phototoxic Cosmetic Chemicals	Reference to Adverse Reaction
DEA methoxycinnamate	can form cancer causing nitrosoamines in sunlight (photo toxin), Ref(150)
digalloyl trioleate	causing photosensitivity, Ref(152, 25,64)
digalloyl trioleate	causing photosensitivity, Ref(152,15,64)
furocoumarin-plus-UVA	phototoxin; reacts with UV radiation to yield genotoxin, Ref(19)
lemon oil (lemon peel oil)	causing photo toxicity, Ref(120)
p-aminobenzoic acid	causing photo sensitivity and contact dermatitis, Ref(120)
PABA (p-aminobenzoic acid)	causing photo sensitivity and contact dermatitis, Ref(120)
psoralen (furocoumarines)	phototoxin; reacts with UV radiation to yield genotoxin, Ref(19)
sulisobenzone (benzophenone-4)	causing photosensitivity, Ref(152, 25,64)
TEA salicylate	can form cancer causing nitrosoamines in sunlight (phototoxin), Ref(150)
ultraviolet (UV)	Hazard: Dangerous to eyes, overexposure causing severe skin burns (sunburn), Ref(149 p.1204)

Protection from UV radiation should be the number one consideration not only when on the beach or skiing in the mountains, but every time we are outdoors. We do not need to damage our skin in order to obtain a rich tan. There are several natural and synthetic substances that are able to block, filter, and reflect dangerous UV radiation when applied to the skin and which do not block those rays that are responsible for gentle tanning. These sunscreens must not only absorb radiation efficiently in the UV-B range but must also fulfill a number of equally important requirements. They should be chemically stable, odorless, and colorless. They must be non-irritating, non-sensitizing, non-allergenic, and non-toxic. In addition, they must show good processability and good solubility in the most important solvents and bases customary in cosmetics. It is not surprising that very few compounds meet all these requirements perfectly for all people. The FDA defines a sunscreen active ingredient as an "ingredient that absorbs at least 85 percent of the light in the UV range at wavelengths from 290 to 320 nanometers, but transmits UV light at wavelengths longer than 320 nanometers. Such agents permit tanning in the average individual and also permit some reddening (erythema) without pain." [9]

In order to measure the effectiveness of a sunscreen a standard called Solar Protection Factor (SPF) was developed in the U.S. and by corresponding standards bodies in Europe. SPF is defined as the ratio of the threshold time until reddening of the skin is observed on your skin with and without a protective substance. A standard (artificial) source of radiation is used for this test. These standards are different for the United States and Europe making the United Stated rating twice the European rating for the same screening effect.

Table 6 Safe Exposure Times to Sun Rays

Day	Minutes of exposure	Acquired natural SPF
1	10	approx. 2.8
2	15	approx. 4.0
3	20	approx. 6.0
4	30	approx. 8.0
5	40	approx. 11.0
6	55	approx. 14.0
7	75	approx. 20.0
Week	Hours of exposure	Acquired natural SPF
1	1-1/4	approx. 20.0
2	4	approx. 60.0
3	10	approx. 140.0

When exposed to unfiltered sunlight, light human skin develops its own natural solar protection factor. If the exposure time is limited each day, with a little patience you can get a rich looking tan without endangering your skin. The average times of exposure each day to reach a healthy tan have been calculated for light skinned people (see Table 6). However, the same exposure time can be lengthened by using a sunscreen. To select the new safe

---

[9]   Proposed rule published by the U.S. Food and Drug Administration, "Sunscreen Drug Products for Over-the-Counter Human Use," 43 Fed. Reg. 38206, August 25, 1978.

exposure time multiply the natural exposure time for each day by the SPF of the preparation and divide by two (in the U.S.). For example, on the first day using a sunscreen preparation SPF 8 you can safely remain in the sun for 10 x 8 / 2 = forty minutes. On the seventh day, the new safe exposure time is five hours. By that time, you should have a beautiful tan without damage to your skin.

The following group of substances and their derivatives have proven to be effective radiation screening agents and are listed in the 43 Fed. Reg. 38206 as safe and effective in sunscreen products. Nevertheless, many of them have been shown to be sensitizers or cause dermatitis in some individuals. Those that are underlined have caused dermatitis or photosensitivity in the past (see Appendix A).

PABA and Derivatives: PABA (p-Aminobenzoic acid), Ethyl dihydroxypropyl PABA (Ethyl 4- (bis(Hydroxypropyl)) Aminobenzoate), Glyceryl PABA (Glyceryl Aminobenzoate), Octyl dimethyl PABA (Padimate O)

Anthranilates: Methyl Anthranilate

Salicylates: Octyl salicylate (2-Ethylhexyl Salicylate), TEA salicylate (Triethanolamine Salicylate)

Cinnamates: DEA-methoxycinnamate (Diethanolamine p-Methoxycinnamate), Octyl methoxycinnamate (Ethylhexyl p-Methoxycinnamate)

Benzophenes: Benzophenone-3 (Oxybenzone), benzophenone-4 (Sulisobenzone), benzophenone-8 (Dioxybenzone)

Others: Cinoxate, Digalloyl trioleate, Octocrylene (2-Ethylhexyl-2-Cyano-3,3-Diphenylacrylate), Homosalate, Red Petrolatum

The FDA proposed a new Code of Federal Regulations (CFR) for sunscreens in 1993. This new regulation is called 21 CFR§700.35 and provides that any product using the term "SUNSCREEN" or the term "SPF", or any SPF value, causes that product to be considered a drug. Similar claims, such as "shields from the sun," "blocks out the rays of the sun," or "protection against UV rays," has the same regulatory effect. Thus, drug related claims will be eliminated from purely cosmetic products, and sunscreen producers will have to meet the more stringent regulations imposed on the drug industry in the future.

My survey showed that about 65 percent of all sunscreen agents listed on product labels in the U.S. are causing allergic and contact dermatitis in some section of the population. As with preservatives, the only way to find out for yourself if a certain sunscreen is right for you is to conduct a patch test.

Colorants

Color is an important part of life itself. Plants use it to lure insects to pollinate and ensure survival of the species. Insects and other animals use it to attract members of the opposite sex for the same purpose. All colors except green help plants to utilize solar energy for life and growth. It is no wonder that for millennia color has played a dominant role in three areas important to man: food, physical appearance, and art.

Archeology and recent history are filled with accounts of the widespread use of color in art and as an additive to cosmetic preparations. The use of color in cosmetics has been documented in Egyptian pyramids and tombs dating back more than 5,000 years. Egyptian women used henna to dye their hair, and kohl (a poisonous antimony compound) to blacken their eyebrows, eyelids, and lashes. In the Old Testament we read that Jezebel "painted her face" (2 Kings 30:9). The ancient Romans painted their faces with lead pigments and dyed their hair. As today, many of the color substances in use were highly toxic.

Until the middle of the last century, colorants for cosmetics and food were produced from natural sources. In the nineteenth century, new synthetic organic color compounds were discovered. They became available in a variety of shades and were stronger and more permanent than natural organic dyes. They were called tar colors and began to be employed immediately in foods and cosmetics without testing for adverse effects. The lavish use of color additives was soon recognized as a threat to the public's health. The history of misuse of colorants during the following 100 years reads like a consumer horror story. The public outcry produced by the publication in 1906 of Upton Sinclair's novel "The Jungle" (a description of the Chicago meat packing industry) and other events of the time finally motivated the U.S. Congress to draft and pass the Food and Drug Act of 1906 which President Theodore Roosevelt signed into law the same year. This was the beginning of a long, drawn-out battle that is still in progress between government and industry over the color certification process.

In 1938 the Food, Drug, and Cosmetic Act was signed into law which outlines the regulatory responsibility of the FDA for colorant materials. In 1939 the FDA recommended 17 coal-tar dyes to be certified, and proposed the creation of three categories that have been adopted for use in the United States. The three categories are:

FD&C Colorants: Colorants certifiable for use in coloring food, drugs, and cosmetics (FD&C) in general.

D&C Colorants: Dyes and pigments considered safe in drugs and cosmetics (D&C) that can be ingested or used in direct contact with mucous membranes.

Ext. D&C Colorants: Colorants not certifiable for use in products intended for ingestion because of their oral toxicity but considered safe for use in products applied to the skin.

During the following years many dyes were added and some were removed after lengthy court battles between the FDA and the cosmetics industry. The last far-reaching revision occurred in 1960 when President Eisenhower signed a law popularly known as the Color Additive Amendments of 1960. It allowed the continued use of existing color additives pending completion of investigations needed to ascertain harmlessness. It also authorized the Secretary of Health, Education, and Welfare to establish limits to the use of colorant materials. A special provision in the law, commonly known as the Delaney clause, specifically directs the Secretary not to list (allow) color additives for any use in food if that colorant can be shown to produce cancer in humans or animals. Since the passage of this amendment no significant additional regulations have been imposed by the FDA in the field of color additives. However, articles continue to appear in the medical literature about adverse effects, including mutagenic and carcinogenic properties of FDA approved colorants. Red dyes (used for blushes) have been shown to promote acne and in June 1993 the FDA had enough evidence to ban FD&C Red No. 3 from cosmetic products on grounds of cytotoxicity.

The subdivision into FD&C, D&C, and Ext. D&C color categories in 1960 reflects the mistaken belief of the time that the skin provides a perfect barrier to topically applied substances, including dyes. In the meantime it has been found that the skin passes significant amounts of dyes and other substances into the body. This can be easily demonstrated by a self-performed test. Just place a small amount of food dye on your forearm. If it cannot be washed off, it has penetrated into the epidermis and deeper. Colorants that have been placed in categories D&C and Ext. D&C have known properties that cause adverse effects. For this reason, the FDA lists "for external use only" as a special restriction while not taking into account the known permeability of skin. In addition, even though most hair coloring agents are toxic, they cannot be found in any FDA category. They can be used without restriction because they are mistakenly presumed not to come in contact with the skin during hair coloring.

The process of certification of a colorant means that each manufacturer must submit to the FDA a sample for each batch of color additive manufactured before shipment. After subsequent analysis, the FDA issues a certificate of acceptance or "certification." Appendix C reflects the latest status on approved colors for foods and cosmetics. You will find that some colorants listed as suitable for food have restrictions placed on them because of potential adverse effects. I strongly recommend avoiding all coloring compounds that are not fit for human consumption (not listed in category FD&C) with the exceptions listed in Appendix C.

Chapter 3

Active Botanical Ingredients

The professional literature for cosmetic formulators lists more than one hundred categories of special ingredients for cosmetic and skin care products. Each of these categories has sometimes over a hundred different entries from which to choose. Over 90 percent of these ingredients are of synthetic origin of which over half have known to cause adverse reactions. None of them have been sufficiently tested for long-term effects on human beings. The ten percent natural ingredients listed represent only a fraction of healthful ingredients that can be used in cosmetic products. The following is a description of some groups that are important as additives to cosmetic preparations and arguments why they should or should not be used.

Plant Materials

No scientist can determine with certainty the size of the plant kingdom. Today's estimates vary between 250,000 and 500,000 species. The relationship between the human species and vegetation has been intimate and vital through the ages. Throughout the development of human cultures man truly has lived with and depended upon green plants. Botany and medicine have been synonymous fields of knowledge throughout history. The shaman or medicine man, usually an accomplished botanist, represents probably the oldest profession in social evolution. Most of the foods and medicines that we now use from the plant kingdom were not discovered by the science of modern societies, but by trial and error over millennia in unlettered cultures.

History

The first known Herbal written more than 5,000 years ago is attributed to Emperor Shen-nung of China whose written and oral traditions identified 239 plant drugs and 365 medicines. He is venerated to this day as a great teacher and medical man by the Chinese people. The Egyptians depicted Thoth, the God of Healing, as pilot of a bark on the Nile. His name is given as Ph-ar-maki, grantor of safety, from which our modern name pharmacy is derived. The Egyptians knowledge of healing herbs was inscribed in tombs and temples more than 4,000 years ago. From the dawn of history many people have faithfully transmitted their medicinal knowledge, mostly by oral tradition, to their posterity.

When Alexander the Great (356-323 B.C.) went to conquer his known world, his aims were to control the East-West trade of gold, gems, precious woods, spices, and medicinal substances. He had a team of researchers accompany his army to learn and record all about the medical knowledge of the conquered nations. Seeds of newly discovered plants were sent to be cultivated in the botanical gardens in Athens. This wealth of knowledge was passed on and has subsequently been used for over two thousand years in Europe and the Orient. The first scientific work of the ancient world that has come down to us is the famous De materia medica libri V that describes more than 600 plants and was written by Pedanius Dioscurides who lived in Greece about 200 A.D. His comprehensive work was copied many times and used as an authoritative work in Europe throughout the Middle Ages and into modern times. From Emperor Shen-nung of China to the physicians and herbalists of today, skin treatments using plant and animal preparations are part of our herbal heritage and history. The ancient civilizations did not treat skin ailments by themselves, but used a holistic approach, since many ailments of the skin have much deeper, systemic, causes. Herbs and other botanical substances described in this book are mainly for topical applications to the skin. Systemic causes of skin disorders are only mentioned peripherally as in the case of vitamin deficiencies.

Scientists all over the world today are in search of new healing substances are using the knowledge of ancient and native herbalists. Research is being done using old records of herbal remedies and oral traditions of natives, like those in South America and Africa. The Mexican government recently conducted a survey of medicinal plants used by various segments of the rural population in Mexico. The survey identified 399 curative products from 237 plants that are used to treat 57 illnesses.[10] Experimental studies confirm some of the healing traditions and open new ways for treatment of illnesses, as in a recent study of an ancient Chinese elixir, Shou Xing Bu Zhi (SXBZ), which confirmed that it is effective in slowing down aging in humans and laboratory animals.[11] Since this book does not focus on plant pharmacology, it describes only those plant materials that can be used in cosmetic products and that have proved beneficial to the skin or hair.

---

[10]   Zamora-Martinez M.C., de-Pascual-Pola C.N., Medicinal plants used in some rural populations of Oaxaca, Puebla and Veracruz, Mexico, Centro de Investigaciones Forestales y Agropecuarias del Distrito Federal, INIFAP, Mexico, *J. Ethnopharmacol.*, 1992 Jan, 35(3), 229-57.

[11]   Chen, J., An experimental study on the anti-senility effects of shou xing bu zhi, Chung. Hsi. I. Chieh. Ho. Tsa. Chi., 1989 Apr, 9 (4):226-7, 198.

Composition

Green plants contain 90 percent water while the water content of wood and bark is only about 50 percent or less. Plants are chemical factories where photosynthesis turns carbon dioxide from the air, water, and minerals into high molecular compounds (cellulose, chitin, lignin, etc.) by means of solar energy. Metabolic action then creates many secondary organic compounds. The value of plants in cosmetics is due to the presence of low molecular weight chemical substances in the plant tissue that are capable of producing a variety of beneficial effects. These active principles are highly complex and their exact chemical nature is still unknown. Active plant principles used in cosmetics most commonly fall into one of six categories: alkaloids, essential oils, glycosides, proteins and enzymes, fats and oils, gums and resins. Each of the first four of these categories will be briefly described. Fats and oils have been described previously in the section on emollients.

Alkaloids: Alkaloids are a diverse group of alkaline compounds containing nitrogen. Many of them have specific effects on the nervous system and many are poisons. With more than 5,000 different known alkaloids, less than 10 percent have been studied in detail. Some examples are cocaine, nicotine, quinine, morphine, mescaline, and caffeine. Since the skin is permeable to a certain extent, alkaloids (especially cocaine derivatives like procaine and benzocaine) have been used as local anesthetics in creams to ease sunburn or other discomforts.

Essential Oils: Many plants have characteristic odors that are mostly pleasant and that stem from special compounds called essential oils, balms, and resins. In their pure form, they are volatile and strong smelling compounds of oil-like consistency that are insoluble in water but are readily soluble in alcohol or hydrocarbon solvents. They are complicated mixtures of organic chemicals. Their economic importance lies in their use in perfumes, cosmetics, medicines, aromatherapy, as well as in food for spices and flavors. The importance of essential oils for skin care, hair care, and aromatherapy is more fully described in the section on essential oils and aromatherapy.

Glycosides: Glycosides are formed in the plant from a saccharide and a non-sugar part (acetal) that can be separated through hydrolysis. The non-sugar compound determines the physiological activity. They form a very important class of drugs of which one of the best known is derived from Foxglove (Digitalis Purpura) and is called digitalis. This drug increases the tone of the cardiac muscle which causes the heart to work more efficiently. It is also used to treat a variety of heart ailments. Another glycoside, called salicin, is extracted from willow bark. The Greeks used extracts of willow bark more than 2,400 years ago to treat pain, gout, and other illnesses. This compound later lead to the development of acetylsalicylic acid (aspirin) that is consumed by Americans at the rate of 50 million tablets daily.

Other glycosides, called saponins, form colloidal dispersions with water. They foam when shaken with water and are compounds similar to our modern surfactants (detergents). They were used as mild cleansing agents for skin before they were displaced by modern synthetic products. Some of the saponin glycosides are useful as hormone precursors. They are said to be mainly responsible for the remarkable properties of ginseng, that will be described in the section on properties of herbs in cosmetics. Some glycosides are similar in structure to animal (and human) steroids and are called sterol glycosides or sterolins. These compounds are used in cosmetic products because of their superior skin softening properties. Another large group of glycosides are called flavonoids that have a variety of medical applications. Flavonoids in Hawthorn, for instance, act as vasodilators and are known to relieve angina pectoris.

Proteins and Enzymes: Proteins are complex organic compounds that are actively present whenever cells metabolize, grow, or divide. Amino acids are the building blocks that form proteins (and other compounds) with the aid of the genetic code DNA (deoxyribonucleic acid). Their molecular size and complexity is enormous. It ranges from several thousands to several millions of atoms per molecule depending upon their function. Plant proteins have recently become important substitutes for animal proteins in cosmetics as moisturizers and in food when formulating vegetarian and kosher products.

Enzymes are an important subgroup of proteins that are also formed inside living cells. They are catalytic substances that make cell metabolism and inter-cellular chemical reaction possible without suffering any changes in the process. Over 2,000 of these substances have been isolated so far, each with a specific task and narrow catalytic capability. Enzymes can be extracted from living organisms and made to perform a variety of important functions outside the cell. They are used in the industry to manufacture cheeses, sourdough bread, beer, wine, and leather. Additionally, they are used to hydrolyze protein, and in a large number of medical applications. Papain is one of the protein-digesting enzymes that is being used in cosmetics for successfully treating age spots, and also as a bleaching agent.

Preparation

Plant materials are used in cosmetics in many ways. The simplest way is to use the actual plant or fresh plant juice and apply it directly to your skin. This would include applying fresh aloe vera juice to your sunburned skin or placing stripes of cucumber on your face for a natural facial. Another way is to prepare fresh plant juices by pressing the actual plant followed by pasteurization for later use. Commercial aloe vera juice is made using this method and is sometimes concentrated by evaporating some of the water. The following are a few methods of extracting plant substances.

Decoction: For plant material that cannot easily be extracted, a certain amount of the plant material, fresh or dried, is boiled with water for a short time. This is similar to an infusion where the plant material is placed in a container and boiling water is added (as in tea).

Distillation: This method is generally used to obtain essential oils which are the odorous principles of the plants. They are volatile oils derived from single botanical species by steam or dry distillation. They serve as raw materials for perfumes, elixirs, spirits, medicinal skin and hair care, and aromatherapeutic applications. True rose oil, which trades for several hundred dollars an ounce, is an example of an essential oil produced by steam distillation.

Extraction: Extractions are usually made from fresh or air dried plant materials using a liquid solvent. This is the form mostly used in cosmetics, except for aloe vera. It is important to know what solvent is used to extract the plant principle. Most plant extractions used in cosmetics have been commercially prepared with propylene glycol. This substance is a good solvent and preservative but has caused dermatitis in about 10 percent of the users and has not been studied for long-term systemic effects. Another solvent is common grain alcohol which is more expensive but is harmless when sufficiently diluted. The extraction of plant oils is briefly described in the section on basic ingredients of creams and lotions.

Absolutes are a special category of materials obtained by extraction. They are made through cold extraction of fragrant plant materials with a gentle solvent like alcohol or butane, and subsequent evaporation of the solvent. This method is used for preparing perfume materials from delicate or heat sensitive plant materials like lilac flowers, lily of the valley, orange flowers, jasmine, and rose. The price of absolutes can reach several hundred dollars per ounce.

Maceration: Herbs containing a high proportion of volatile oils and mucilage are best steeped in cold water for several hours. This process is usually designed for immediate use.

Plant products obtained by the above processes can be processed further and separated into more basic components. An example is mucilage, which occurs in many land and sea plants. -One form of sea algae (laminaria digitata) yields the raw material for the production of alginates that play an important role in the food and cosmetics industry (ice cream, cheese, cosmetic thickeners). Pure natural alkaloids are also produced by further processing plant extracts for medical purposes. The production of pure phospholipids (PC and PE) from raw soybean oil is another example of separating single components from plant extracts for a special purpose.

Botanical Substances for Cosmetics

To take advantage of a new customer trend, many cosmetic companies are including herbal extracts and essential oils in their products. My survey showed that most of the herbal extracts sold as raw material use propylene glycol as a solvent, which is causing side effects in many users. In addition, these products contain other harmful ingredients that can certainly eliminate any useful effect of the herbal principles. Another concern is dosage of herbal principles. A minimum concentration is needed for a particular herb to have an effect on skin or hair. Judging from the lack of color in most preparations, the concentrations of herbal principles are too low to have any effect. This may be a good thing since I found that about 40 percent of all botanical ingredients listed on cosmetic product labels in the U.S. have caused adverse reactions in the past. However, a large number of plant extracts and essential oils cause little or no side effects and are very beneficial to your skin and general health. The attributes for some of the most beneficial herbs and essential oils for skin and hair care are described below and a summary is provided in Tables 7 and 8 (see pages 64 and 81).

Herbs for Cosmetics

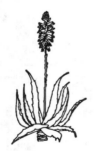

Fig. 31 *Aloe (aloe vera)*

Aloe (*aloe vera*): The aloe is a perennial plant found wild in East and South Africa and also cultivated in the West Indies and in southern United States. Modern medical reports concerning the medicinal value of aloe leaves began to appear over 50 years ago. Patients suffering from facial x-ray burns were healed in a short time and without suffering scars when treated with fresh aloe juice. Many human and animal tests since have confirmed the remarkable properties of this plant. In domestic medicine the use of aloe as an aid to relieve burning, itching, minor cuts, and first and second degree burns is spreading rapidly. The main active principle is believed to be aloin, a C-glycoside manufactured by the plant. The cosmetic industry has become the main user of aloe vera because of its healing and soothing, antibacterial, and moisturizing qualities. Recent studies indicate that aloe vera gel has the ability to enhance or accelerate cell growth in the skin. It is a frequent ingredient in sunscreen and after-sun preparations, creams, lotion and wash substances.

Althea (*althea officinalis*): see marsh mallow

Burdock (*arctium lappa*): Burdock is a biennial plant found in the northern United States, Europe and Asia. The thistle-like fruit heads along with their hooked prickles cling to almost anything. The medicinal properties of this plant are concentrated in both the root and leaves. Its outstanding effects on the human skin have been valued in places such as Chile, China, India, Canada and Russia. It has been used as a remedy against skin cancer. Homeopaths prescribe the tincture of the fresh root to heal acne and eczema, and herbalists praise it as an excellent remedy for all skin diseases. Oil extracts produced from the root and plant is said to restore the smoothness of skin and to promote hair growth. No wonder that the cosmetic industry is starting to use burdock extracts and oils in skin care and scalp preparations. The plant contains essential oil (0.2%), abundant inulin, and antibiotic substances.

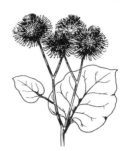

Fig. 32 *Burdock (arctium lappa)*

Chamomile (*matricaria chamomilla*): Chamomile is a Southern European annual plant found wild along roadsides, in fields, and cultivated in gardens. This is a versatile medicinal herb with a wide range of uses, both internal and external. The essential oil that is distilled from the leaves and flowers is among the few essential oils that do not irritate the skin but have counter-irritant, antiinflammatory, antiseptic, and anodyne properties. Extracts of the flowery parts are used in a variety of creams and lotions, bath oils and foam baths, shampoos and sun-burn preparations and for sensitive or allergy- prone skin. Its effectiveness as a skin care agent is partly attributed to azulene, chamazulene, and bisabolol.

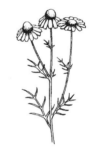

Fig. 33 *Chamomile (matricaria chamomilla)*

Comfrey (*symphytum officinalis*): Comfrey is a perennial plant common in moist meadows and other moist places in the United States and Europe. This herb has been used for centuries in Europe to heal wounds and broken bones. In addition, it is reported to be effective against several types of cancer, including skin cancer. The active principle that has been isolated in comfrey is allantoin that is today manufactured from different sources for medical and cosmetic purposes. During the first World War, Allantoin was found to contribute to the speedy healing of large wounds. The whole plant is no longer used because it also contains large amounts of tannin and lasiocarpine, both of which have been implicated to cause cancer in laboratory animals.

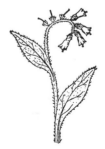

Fig. 34 *Comfrey (symphytum officinalis)*

Allantoin is used today in its pure form as a valuable additive to cosmetic creams and lotions, sun screens, and after-sun preparations.

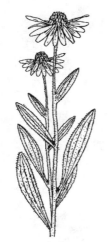

Echinacea (*echinacea augustifolia*): This native herbaceous plant grows from the prairie states eastward to Pennsylvania. The therapeutic value of this herb was well known to the AmericanIndians who used it for treating wounds. Modern research found that the root contains a substance, echinacoside, that is antimicrobial. In addition, extracts of the plant have been shown to marshal effectively the body's immune system and increase the resistance against infections. It is used internally as a blood purifier and in cosmetics as an additive to creams and lotions to speed healing of skin conditions caused by acne, eczema, and other problems.

Fig. 35 *Echinacea (echinacea augustifolia)*

Gotu Kola (*centella asiatica, hydrocotyle asiatica*): Gotu Kola is a small creeping herb that grows wild in India and the islands of the Indian Ocean. Species grown in certain jungle districts of the Eastern Tropics are believed to contain remarkable rejuvenating properties and Gotu Kola is one of the reported "elixirs of life," similar to Ginseng. It is a grazing crop for elephants and is described by the natives as representing a whole "apothecary shop" curing a variety of illnesses, including cancers. It is eaten raw, or cooked, and sometimes used as a tea. It has been shown to help mice to overcome fatigue-stress situations and increase their vitality. Extracts of Gotu Kola are said to be useful for stressed skin, to heal wounds, dermatitis, inflammations, and are a valued skin tonic. The composition of this herb is not well researched but it is believed that certain glycosides and saponins are responsible for its properties.

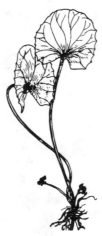

Fig. 36 *Gotu kola (centella asiatica)*

Ginseng (*panax ginseng*): Asiatic ginseng is a small perennial plant that grows in the damp woodlands of Manchuria and is primarily cultivated in Korea. The aromatic root commonly grows to a length of two feet. For more than 5,000 years the Chinese have steadfastly maintained that ginseng has great influence in curing a variety of ills. It would be foolish to suppose that more than 150 generations of Chinese were founding their faith in ginseng on sheer superstition. They would have discarded this belief long ago if it did not produce genuine results. From all the evidence collected, ginseng acts as a true reactivator and rejuvinator. Chinese men who can afford to use ginseng are able to retain their virility as long as they live and to procreate children through and beyond the age of seventy. Unfortunately, ginseng's high reputation in the Orient ensures that the wild plant will remain extremely rare.

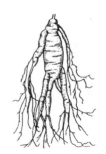

Fig. 37 *Ginseng (panax ginseng)*

Research to determine the actual composition and active principles is ongoing. Recent studies indicate that polysaccharides in ginseng have anti-inflammatory properties. It was also found that ginseng activates cell metabolism and prolongs the life span of human cells. It definitely influences the hormone balance and increases cell proliferation. It is for these reasons that it hasbecome a prized additive to tonics, and creams and lotions to revitalize stressed skin. You will find ginseng extracts in antiwrinkle and antiaging creams, and products for maintaining a healthy skin. The FDA steadfastly refuses to acknowledge these valuable properties of ginseng and has been known to seize products containing ginseng due to "unfounded claims" professed on the label.

Horsetail or Shave grass (*equisetum arvense*): Horsetail is a perennial plant common in moist loamy and sandy soil all over North America and Eurasia. Its uses as a medicinal herb go back to Roman times when it was used to heal wounds and stop bleeding. In addition, the herbalist Kneipp recommends the use of horsetail extracts to heal tumors and cancer. It is also an effective remedy to treat psoriasis, dandruff, eczema, and similar skin conditions. Europeans praise its ability to effectively reduce the swelling of eyelids and its anticellulite properties. Horsetail contains 5 to 8 percent of silicic acid and a number of glycosides that are believed to be the active ingredients.

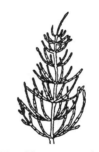

Fig. 38 *Horsetail (equisetum arvense)*

Mallow or Blue mallow (*malva sylvestris, rotundifolia*): Mallow is an annual or perennial plant found in wastelands and fields. It is consistently cultivated in Europe and sparingly in the United States. Blue mallow has a long history of use by herbalists for various skin conditions. It has antiinflammatory properties and has been used as a wash to relieve discomfort due to dry eyelids and dry mucous membranes. It is said to control oily skin and is used

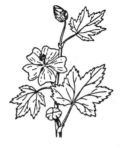

Fig. 39 *Mallow (malva sylvestris)*

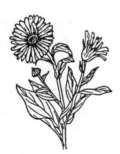

Fig. 40 *Marigold (calendula officinalis)*

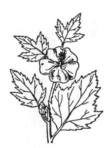

Fig. 41 *Marsh mallow (althea officinalis)*

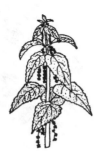

Fig. 42 *Nettle (urtica dioica)*

to help with allergic skin reactions and comedogenic conditions. It is a frequent ingredient in face creams and lotions for sensitive skin. It is also found in skin tonics to counteract allergies, irritations, and dryness. The effectiveness of blue mallow is believed to be due to its high content of a special mucilage (mucin) that is soothing to mucous membranes and an emollient for inflammation.

Marigold (*calendula officinalis*): Marigold is an annual garden plant that is seldom found in the wild. The flowery parts of this plant have been used for centuries in Europe to prepare salves for the healing of skin ailments and wounds. It is antiinflammatory and has been reported to be effective in treating skin cancer as well. Most recent investigations confirm that the flower has medicinal properties and promotes healing of skin tissue. Marigold extracts are used in cosmetics as additives to sunscreen and after-sun preparations, although some adverse skin reactions have been reported in the medical literature.

Marsh mallow or Althea (*althea officinalis*): Althea is a perennial plant that grows in damp meadows and wet places and is also cultivated as a medicinal plant. Althea has been used since pre-historic time and its name is derived from Greek, meaning healing. It has antiinflammatory properties and has been used as a wash to relieve discomfort due to dry eyelids and dry mucous membranes. It is said to control oily skin and is used to help with allergic skin reactions and comedogenic conditions.

Nettle (*urtica dioica*): Nettle is a perennial plant native to the woods and meadows in North America and Europe. It was immortalized in the 15th century when the famous German painter, Albrecht Dürer, painted an angel carrying a stinging nettle into God's presence. The plant has been highly praised as a blood purifier that is said to clear skin conditions when taken internally as tea. Its ability to increase micro circulation of the skin makes it a frequent component of preparations to treat thinning hair. It is said to stimulate metabolism and is used in lotions for treatment of dark circles around the eyes. The fresh plant contains large amounts of vitamin C, glucoquinine, and nettle toxins. The nettle toxins completely decompose upon drying or boiling.

Plantain (*plantago major, lanceolata*): Plantain is a perennial plant that inhabits meadows, roadside, and agricultural lands in the eastern United States and Europe. This tough little plant is mentioned in the earliest herbals in England and on the European continent. It is said to heal many skin ailments, tone the skin, and is indispensable to healing of wounds. It is used in cosmetic preparations because of its soothing properties for irritated skin and protection of mucous membranes, ability to contract organic tissues (astringent) and reduce oil secretion of the skin. Plantain contains the glycoside aucubin, tannins, and mucilage as active principles.

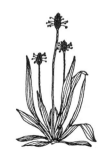

Fig. 43 *Plantain (plantago major)*

Shave grass (*equisetum arvense*): See Horsetail.

St. Johnswort (*hypericum perforatum*): St. Johnswort is a shrubby perennial plant commonly found in dry, gravelly soils, fields, and sunny places in the Northern Hemisphere. Its use dates back many centuries in Europe where it has been used for a variety of purposes including healing wounds. St. Johnswort oil is made from lipid extraction of the herb. Its value in cosmetics is based on its soothing and antiinflammatory properties. It is used in creams and lotions for sensitive skin. It is a valued healing agent for burns, is used in sunscreen and after-sun preparations, and is also recommended as a skin tightener. The active principles in St. Johnswort are essential oils, hyperin, rutin, hypericin, tannin, and choline.

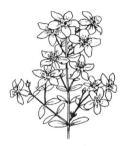

Fig. 44 *St.Johnswort (hypericum perforatum)*

Witch hazel (*hamamelis virginiana*): Witch hazel is a deciduous shrub or small tree which grows in damp woods from Georgia to Nova Scotia. North American Indians taught the early settlers about this medicinal herb which they used to cure inflamed skin, in particular inflamed eyes due to infections. Its astringent properties have made it a frequent additive to sensitive skin preparations such as toners and after-shave lotions. The principle active substances are hamamelitannin, choline, and saponins.

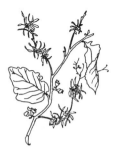

Fig. 45 *Witch hazel (hamamelis virginiana)*

Table 7 Herbal Ingredients for Skin and Hair Care

Herb	Remarks
allantoin	active principle in comfrey (symphytum officinalis), has proven healing properties; used in after-sun preparation, anti-acne and clarifying lotions.
aloe (aloe vera)	reported to heal many kinds of skin ailments including burns (also sun burns) and cancer (Ref. 147).
alpha-bisabolol	active principle in chamomile (matricaria chamomilla), counter-irritant, antiinflammatory, non-allergenic; used in sensitive skin preparations, anti-acne products
alpha hydroxy acids	naturally occurring fruit acids; moisturizing, toning, peeling; used in moisturizing creams and peeling products that do not require scrubbing.
althea extract (marsh mallow)	high in mucilage. Reported to heal eczema and dermatitis; used in before- and after-sun preparations, and damaged skin products (Ref. 148). Althea means healing in Greek.
balm (melissa officinalis)	used in toners and sensitive skin products, and counter irritant preparations, (Ref. 120). For bath oils and foam baths.
bilberry (vaccinium myrtillus)	anti-inflammatory. Sensitive skin preparations. Used in mouth wash to control gingivitis (Ref. 142).
birch (betula pendula)	regulates sebum production. Reported to heal sebaceous cyst (Ref. 141). Used in hair loss preparations (Ref. 142).
bisabolol	see alpha-bisabolol
burdock (arctium lappa)	astringent; antibacterial, antidandruff; sebum regulator; for hair and scalp treatment; anti-acne preparations, ref(142); reported effective against certain skin cancers and tumors, ref(147)
calendula	see marigold
chamomile (matricaria chamomilla)	antimicrobial; anti-inflammatory preparations (puffed eyes), sun and after sun preparations, bath preparations, ref(147); can cause allergic dermatitis in creams, ref(120)

Herb	Remarks
comfrey (symphytum officinalis)	contains allantoin, a proven wound healing and skin conditioning agent but can cause skin irritations, ref(120)
cornflower (centaurea cyanus)	causing allergy and photosensitivity, ref(120)
cucumber (cucumis sativus)	astringent; for facial preparations
echinacea (echinacea angustifolia)	sun and after sun preparations; severely damaged skin products
flavonoids	glycosides that have skin toning properties; used in products that strengthen fragile capillaries and tone the skin
garlic (allium sativum)	used for anti-bacterial preparations and acne products; reported to heal certain skin cancers, ref(142); Caution! fresh garlic juice can cause severe burns
ginseng (panax ginseng)	stimulant; anti-wrinkle, anti-aging creams and lotions, ref(143); reported to prolong cell life, ref(147); linked to vaginal bleeding, ref(57)
gotu kola (centella asiatica, hydrocotyle asiatica)	anti-wrinkle, anti-aging products, ref(143), cleans and heals skin ailments, including cancer, ref(147)
hops (humulus lupulus)	anti-stress preparations; antimicrobial; preventive aging preparations; dark circle treatment; reported to cause dermatitis in some individuals, ref(147)
horse tail (equisetum arvense)	wrinkle treatment, anticellulite products; reduces swelling of eyelids, ref(147)
horse chestnut (aesculus hippocastanum)	anti-inflammatory (puffy eyes); anti-blotches - fragile capillary treatment; sensitive skin treatment; after sun treatment, ref(147)
indian cress (tropaeolum majus)	broad spectrum antibacterial and antifungal agent; weak irritant that increases circulation; used in thinning hair preparations; preventive aging;

Herb	Remarks
ispaghul extract (seed of plantago)	all parts of this plant have healing and antiinflammatory properties, ref(147); stimulates micro circulation
mallow (blue mallow, malva sylvestries)	antiinflammatory and antiallergenic agent; removes discomfort due to dry eyelids and dry muscous membranes and is used to condition sensitive skin
marsh mallow (althea officinalis)	high in mucilage, reported to heal eczema and dermatitis; used in before and after sun preparations, and damaged skin products ref(148) (althea means healing in Greek)
marigold (calendula officinalis)	reported to be effective against cancer of connective tissues (sarcoma), ref(147), also causing irritant dermatitis from plant and tincture, ref(120)
nettle (urtica dioica)	see stinging nettle
plantain (plantago)	astringent and soothing agent; plantain has been used for millenia to tone the skin and heal many skin ailments including allergies
sage (salvia officinalis)	astringent and antiperspirant/ deodorant agent; essential oil increases micro circulation; contains estrogenic substances; effective in stimulating hair growth, ref(147)
scotch pine (pinus sylvestris)	skin tonic; essential oil increases microcirculation; fragrance component; for use in refreshing bath oils and foam bath
St. Johnswort (hypericum perforatum)	astringent agent, antibiotic (preservative) agent; antiinflammatory agent; sensitive skin preparations (blotches); sun and after sun products; essential oil recommended as skin tightener, ref(147)
stinging nettle (urtica dioica)	vasodilator; increases microcirculation; thinning hair preparations, ref(147); preventive aging and dark circle treatment products
witch hazel (hamamelis virginiana)	astringent and antiinflammatory agent; reported to heal skin and eye inflammations due to infections

There is an almost endless list of substances that can be extracted from plants that are and have been used for medicinal purposes and general well-being of man. You can find a description of them in books on the subject of Medical Botany and in Pharmacopoeia. A few of them are very popular and are used in many cosmetic products today. There is a whole industry that produces exotic plant extracts and purified compounds derived from plants and animals that are offered to the cosmetic formulator for specialty products. I will give only a short description of those you may find on the ingredient labels of cosmetic products.

Alginates: The over ten thousand members of the algae plant family can have structures that vary from single celled entities to plants that extend over several hundred feet in the ocean and grow to become the largest plants on earth. It is estimated that algae in the ocean manufacture more hydrocarbons through photosynthesis than all land plants combined. Because they live in the water they do not need supporting structures like cellulose and lignin. Instead, they contain slimy substances inside and outside their individual cells that support the life processes in the water. These substances play an important role as raw materials for the food industry and cosmetics. They are a mixture of many substances, chemically called polysaccharides, that have strong gel-like properties. They form giant molecules consisting of chains of atoms (over 200,000) that can form a stiff gel at a concentration of only one percent. The salts of the alginic acid, called alginates, are water soluble, do not gel, but form viscous solutions. They are used to make dental impressions, stabilize ice cream, form emulsions, as suspending agents in soft drinks and as emollients and thickeners in cosmetic creams and lotions. They are colorless and tasteless, impart a slippery feeling, and form a thin protective film on the surface of the skin or hair.

Allantoin: Comfrey (symphytum officinalis) has been used for hundreds of years in folk medicine as a remedy for healing wounds and mending bones. During World War I it was found that serious wounds healed speedily when treated with comfrey, even when infested with maggots. Later, scientists isolated a substance from comfrey called allantoin which is responsible for the healing action. It is still used topically to stimulate healing of wounds and ulcers. Allantoin also occurs in many other plants like cauliflower, sugar beets, potatoes, chestnuts, and others. It is produced commercially mainly by synthesis from uric acid. Allantoin is a valued ingredient in all types of creams and lotions, especially in after-sun lotions, to repair sunburns, clarifying lotions, and any preparation where skin repair is important. It is used in anti-acne preparations and is said to help obtain a soft and supple skin. No adverse effects have been reported from its use.

Alpha-Bisabolol: Camomile (matricaria chamomilla) teas and extracts have been known for centuries to be antiinflammatory, antimicrobial, and anti-spasmodic. The essential oil extracted from Camomile contains Bisabolol, one of the active principles of the plant, that has been successfully employed externally as a counterirritant liniment for hemorrhoids, skin and mucous membrane inflammations, and sores. Bisabolol is also found in many other plants and is produced commercially. It is non-allergenic and has antiseptic properties as well. It takes about 24 hours until counterirritant and antiinflammatory results are observable when applied topically to the skin. Alpha- bisabolol is used in creams and lotions for sensitive skin, after-sun lotions and other applications when counterirritant and antiinflammatory properties in a preparation are sought.

Alpha Hydroxy Acids: These are the newest additions of biological ingredients for skin and hair care. Alpha hydroxy acids occur naturally in fruits, such as apples, grapefruit, black currants, bilberries, and others, as well as in animals. Chemically they are called glycolic acid (from sugar cane), citric acid (from citrus fruits and red fruits), malic acid (from apples and red fruits), lactic acid (occurring in animal tissues), and others. Lactic acid is also present in the horny layer of the human skin. It is hygroscopic and therefore a natural moisturizer. These organic acids, when applied topically, have a twofold effect on the skin. In small concentrations they act as moisturizers and have a plasticising effect. In larger amounts they facilitate desquamation of dead skin cells (peeling effect). This exfoliating activity is softer than mechanical peeling, which better suits the more fragile skin of the face. Alpha hydroxy acids -containing creams and lotions are offered as moisturizers, for re-activation of dull and tired skin and in peeling products. The FDA is now in the process of studying the potential adverse effects of alpha hydroxy acids and their derivatives in cosmetic products. The results should be available by the end of 1994.

Flavonoids: Flavonoids belong to the family of glycosides and received their name from the yellow extract of the dyers oak containing the flavonoid quercetin (lat. flavus = yellow). Flavonoids have long been known to have medicinal properties. Some, like those contained in hawthorn, have a vasodilator effect and are used internally to relieve pains due to agina pectoris. Others have been shown to prevent the breaking of fragile capillaries, including those of the skin, and to decrease the permeability of certain tissues. They have been recommended for toning the skin and for increasing the oxygen metabolism. Some plants which contain flavonoids are birch, blackthorn, elder, fo-ti-tieng, ginkgo, hawthorn, linden, and others. Any cosmetic preparation containing flavonoids, or other active plant principles, can change the structure of the skin and, according to FDA regulations, may have to treated as a drug.

Essential Oils and Fragrances for Cosmetics

From the dawn of history until modern times, fragrances and flavors have played an important part in the history of mankind. Fragrances have been perceived as a manifestation of divinity on the earth and were used in sacred ceremonies in the temples of old. The Veda, the most sacred book of India and one of the oldest known books, mentions more than 700 different fragrance materials for medicinal and religious practices, such as cinnamon, spikenard, myrrh, and sandalwood. The Egyptians used aromatic materials in their temple for ritual purposes and embalming. Subsequently the practice spread to Israel, Greece, Rome, and the entire Mediterranean world. After a long period of barbarism and general decline of knowledge in Europe during the Dark Ages, revival came from the Arabic countries with the advent of Islam. They revived the art of medicine and perfumery and perfected the techniques to obtain refined products. During the Renaissance, the use of essential oil expanded into perfumery and cosmetics. Advances in the art of distillation made it possible to produce elixirs, balms, scented waters, and fragrant oils. Some of these products, like the famous Cologne water, are still produced today. The main ingredients were alcohol, essential oils, and absolutes.

Essential oils and fragrance materials extracted from flowers are mixtures of hundreds of very complex organic chemicals. Modern chemistry has been able, to a large extent, to identify these compounds and to find more inexpensive ways to produce them from either more abundant plant material or by chemical synthesis. Research on perfume composition is now done by specialized fragrance chemists who have hundreds of chemicals at their disposal to recreate any odor from lily-of-the-valley to musk. However, they are not completely successful in creating such well-known scents as jasmine and rose, so that a small percentage of the real natural extracts is still being used in expensive perfumes. Natural and artificial perfumes and fragrance materials are among the most frequent sensitizers and causes of allergic dermatitis in cosmetic products. Of the almost 900 fragrance chemicals listed by Nater (Reference 152), more than 15 percent are known to cause adverse reactions on skin while the rest have not been sufficiently tested. Since a fragrance can contain up to a hundred or more different compounds, the chances that one of them will cause problems is very high. The safest way for the consumer to avoid immediate skin problems due to fragrances, or other cosmetic preparations, is to conduct a patch test (see section on Skin Care).

Properties of Essential Oils for Cosmetics

The following is a description of a few essential oils and their beneficial properties for skin and hair care. A summary of their properties is provided in Table 8 (page 81).

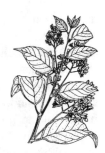

Fig. 46 *Benzoin (styrax benzoin)*

Benzoin Oil (*styrax benzoin*): Benzoin is a natural, balsamic resin that is exuded from a small tree grown in Sumatra and Malaya. This resin is almost completely soluble in alcohol and its composition varies according to growing area. The Siam benzoin consists primarily of benzoates, while resins from Sumatra contain cinnamates of coniferyl alcohol, cinnamyl alcohol, benzoresinol, and other compounds. Both types contain vanillin, which gives them a characteristic odor. Oil of Benzoin is antiseptic, deodorizing, and has a calming influence on itching skin. It is used to heal and soothe inflamed, irritated, and cracked areas of the skin due to environmental (contact dermatitis) influences. The oil is extensively used in perfumery and valued for its rich sweetness and deep balsamic note.

Bois de Rose Oil (*aniba roseodora*): See Rosewood oil.

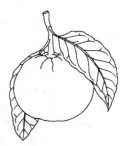

Fig. 47 *Bergamot (citrus bergamia)*

Bergamot Oil (*citrus bergamia*): The bergamot tree grows almost exclusively in a narrow coastal strip in Calabria, Italy. Bergamot oil is produced by cold expression from the peels of the bergamot fruit. It is a green or olive green liquid and consists mainly of linalylacetate, linalool, and methyl-anthranilate. The effect of the oil on the skin is antiseptic, astringent, deodorizing, and healing. It is helpful in controlling dandruff, seborrheic conditions, some forms of herpes (shingles), including genital herpes. It is an antiperspirant and reduces overproduction of sebum. It is therefore used in products to control oily skin and hair as well as common acne. After treatment with bergamot oil, or perfumes containing bergamot oil, direct exposure to sunlight must be avoided since it increases the sensitivity of the skin to ultraviolet light and promotes tanning and sunburn. The oil is extensively used in the perfume industry. It has an extremely rich, sweet-fruity initial odor that is followed by a still more characteristic oily-herbaceous and somewhat balsamic note.

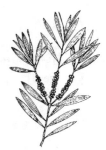

Fig. 48 *Cajeput (melaleuca leucadendron)*

Cajeput Oil (*melaleuca leucadendron*): Cajeput oil is steam distilled from the fresh leaves and twigs of the Cajeput tree (meaning white wood) which is grown in the Philippines, and on the islands between Australia and Malaysia. This thin oil can be colorless, pale yellow, greenish or turquoise and is highly valued among the native people for its medicinal qualities. It is a popular household remedy in the Far East and used for colds, throat diseases, pains, headaches and similar problems. Its main ingredients are cineol, pinene, and terpineol and it is similar in composition to eucalyptus oil. The oil is antiseptic, anodyne and is used to relieve painful skin inflammations. It has been successfully used to treat acne and dandruff and for preventive hair loss preparations. Cajeput oil has a powerful, fresh, eucalyptus-like, camphoraceous odor and a characteristic almost fruity-sweet after note.

Cedarwood Oil (*cedrus virginiana*): The oil is distilled from sawdust and other waste wood of the Virginian Cedar which is found growing wild all over the southeastern United States. It is a pale yellow to slightly orange colored liquid. Its main constituents are cedrene, a sesquiterpene, cedrol, and cedrenol (which give the oil its characteristic cedar odor), borneol, limonene, camphor, and thujon. It is an oil well suited for skin care; it is antiseptic, astringent, and calming and is found in products that treat oily skin, acne, inflammations, eczema, dermatitis, and itching skin. It is used for hair care as well, especially for oily hair, dandruff and psoriasis conditions. It is used as a deodorant and has insect repelling qualities. It is also used extensively in the perfume industry. The odor of Virginian cedar oil is oily-woody and almost sweet, mild and pleasant, and somewhat balsamic.

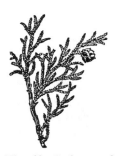

Fig. 49 *Cederwood (cedrus virginiana)*

Chamomile Oil, Blue (*matricaria chamomilla*): The oil is steam distilled from the true chamomile plant which grows all over Europe. The freshly distilled oil is deep blue and turns brown after long storage. The blue color is due to a compound called azulene, which has dermatological value. The main components are butyl, amyl, and hexyl esters of tiglic and angelic acids and bisabolol. Together with azulene, they are highly effective in clearing inflammations and in hastening the healing process of skin conditions. Chamomile oil causes narrowing of blood vessels (vasoconstriction) of the skin. It is a very expensive oil and is used mainly for medicinal purposes. Its odor is first intensely sweet and herbaceous coumarin-like with a fresh fruity undertone, and later becomes pleasant sweet tobacco-like and warm.

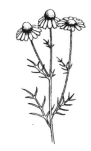

Fig. 50 *Chamomile, blue (matricaria chamomilla)*

Chamomile Oil, Roman (*anthemis nobilis*): The plant is botanically related to the true chamomile mentioned above but looks more like a wild chrysanthemum. It is cultivated in several European countries. The oil is produced by steam distillation and is a pale blue liquid when fresh. It is very similar in composition to the German chamomile described above. It is antiseptic, astringent and has healing properties for dermatitis, eczema, acne, and rashes. It is especially effective in treating sensitive, dry, and inflamed skin and acts as a vasoconstrictor. It is antiallergenic and has been successfully used to treat fragile capillaries. Roman

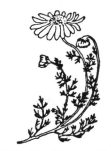

Fig. 51 *Chamomile, roman (anthemis nobilis)*

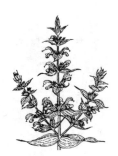

Fig. 52 *Clary sage (salvia sclarea)*

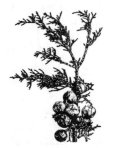

Fig. 53 *Cypress (cupressus sempervirens)*

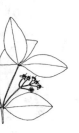

Fig. 54 *Eucalyptus (eucalyptus globulus)*

chamomile oil has a sweet-herbaceous, somewhat fruity-warm and tea leaf-like odor with little tenacity. It is used sparingly in the perfume industry because of its high price and is preferred over the German chamomile oil because of its lighter color.

Clary Sage Oil (*salvia sclarea*): Clary sage is a tall perennial plant that is often cultivated in gardens and originated in countries bordering the Mediterranean. Clary sage oil is steam distilled from the flowering tops and leaves of the plant. It is a colorless to pale yellow or pale olive-colored liquid. Its main constituents are linalool and linalyl acetate. It also contains plant substances that are said to have an estrogen-like effect. Clary sage oil is deodorizing and has a vitalizing effect on scalp, is effective for dandruff control, and in peeling dead skin from the epidermis. Its odor is first sweet-herbaceous, tenacious, and soft that becomes balsamic and tea-like upon drying out.

Cypress Oil (*cupressus sempervirens*): The cypress tree originated in the eastern Mediterranean countries and can now be found all over southern Europe and northern Africa. The oil is distilled from the leaves (needles) and twigs of the evergreen cypress tree. It is a pale yellow, pale olive-greenish, or almost colorless liquid. The main constituents of the oil are mono terpenes, pinene, camphene, and other materials that give it the characteristic odor. It is used in natural cosmetics as an astringent, or deodorant, and to treat varicose veins. It is a vasoconstrictor and has a tightening effect on the skin in general. It is used to treat oily skin and is effective in treating and deodorizing sweating feet. Cypress oil is also an insect repellant. The odor is sweet-balsamic, yet refreshing and reminiscent of pine needle oil. Later, a unique fragrance of tenacious sweetness develops.

Eucalyptus Oil (*eucalyptus globulus*): The homeland of the eucalyptus tree is the island of Tasmania and the tree is now planted all over the world in temperate and semi-tropical areas. The essential oil is steam distilled from the fresh and partly dried leaves. It is colorless and contains mainly cineol. The antibacterial properties and its use to disinfect and heal the bronchial passages are well known. It is a mild skin irritant and is used as a rubefacient and also for acute inflammations, including herpes. The oil is said to have an estrogen effect on the human body and has wound-healing properties through fostering formation of new tissues. It is also used as an insect repellant and in the cosmetic industry as a soap perfume.

Fennel Oil (*foeniculum vulgare*): The plant is only cultivated in southern Europe and probably originated in Malta. Fennel oil is steam distilled from the crushed seeds of the plant. It is a pale yellow or almost colorless liquid. It consists mainly of anethole, limonene, and phellandrene and some estrogen-like substances. It is a diuretic and contains ingredients that are antiinflammatory and have a tightening effect on the skin. It is used as massage oil to strengthen muscle tone and increase the elasticity of connecting tissues and of the skin. It is often an ingredient in antiwrinkle, antiaging skin, and cellulitis products. Its antibacterial properties make it a valuable ingredient for natural toothpastes and mouthwashes. Fennel oil has a somewhat sharp and warm-camphoraceous odor, initially earthy, but later on sweet, anisic, and spicy.

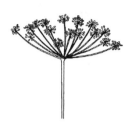

Fig. 55 *Fennel (foeniculum vulgare)*

Fir Oil (*abies sibirica*): There are at least ten different species of plants that are used to produce fir oils, although some are derived from pine trees. Abies sibirica is a fir and yields a true fir needle oil, although its commercial name is Siberian pine needle oil. The tree grows in abundance in the northeastern parts of Russia and in various European countries. It is a colorless to very pale yellow or pale olive-yellow liquid. It has a high content of bornyl acetate, several terpenes, pinene, and phellandrene. The oil has several outstanding qualities. It is a strong antiseptic and is used like eucalyptus to disinfect and heal inflammations of bronchial passages. It has good deodorizing qualities that are used for foot creams to control excessive sweating. As a component of bath oils it soothes rheumatic complaints and it has been shown to relieve stress, nervousness, and mental exhaustion. Its odor is refreshing balsamic with a powerful forest odor, and a peculiar fruity-balsamic undertone.

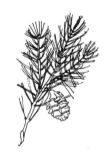

Fig. 56 *Fir (abies sibirica)*

Frankincense Oil (*boswellia carterii*): These small trees originated in the mountainous areas of western India, southern Arabia, and northeastern Africa. Oil of frankincense (also called oil of olibanum) is produced from the raw resinoid by steam distillation. It has a pale yellow or pale amber-greenish color. The Egyptians used frankincense thousands of years ago for skin care. It's cell regenerative and astringent properties make it a valuable skin care ingredient today. It is used in preparations for aging skin and wrinkle treatments as well as for rough and dry skin and to heal inflammations. The odor of frankincense oil is strongly diffusive, fresh-terpeney, reminiscent of unripe apples with a rich, sweet-woody, balsamic undertone.

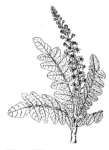

Fig. 57 *Frankincense (boswellia carterii)*

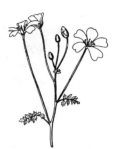

Fig. 58 *Geranium (pelargonium graveolens)*

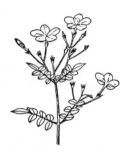

Fig. 59 *Jasmine (jasminum officinale)*

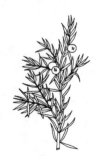

Fig. 60 *Juniper (juniperus communis)*

Geranium Oil (*pelargonium graveolens*): Over half of the world production of geranium oil comes from La Reunion, a small island in the Indian Ocean. The oil is distilled from leaves and branches of the small plant. It is a thin clear liquid and its main ingredients are citronellol, geraniol, terpineol, linalool, terpenes, esters, and eugenol. Its properties are antiseptic, astringent, deodorizing, toning, and antiinflammatory. It stimulates the lymphatic system. It equalizes sebum production in the skin and is highly recommended for oily skin and acne. Other applications are strengthening of the connective tissues of the skin, treatment of cellulitis, seborrheic conditions, acne, eczema, and inflammations. It has been successfully used to treat herpes and fungal problems and certain cancers. The odor of geranium oil is rich sweet-rosy and powerful, with a pronounced fruity-minty undertone.

Jasmine Absolute (*jasminum officinale*): The Jasmine flower originated in the mountainous regions of northwest India and has been known and used for thousands of years. Morocco and Italy are the main producers of the raw material from which the absolute is produced. Jasmine absolutes are made through cold extraction of fragrant plant materials (concrete). The price of jasmine absolutes can reach several hundred dollars per ounce. The fragrant material is a dark orange, somewhat viscous liquid. It is antiseptic, used to tone the skin, and has antiinflammatory properties which make it especially suited for dry and sensitive skin. In general it acts as an aphrodisiac and it is said that a bath using jasmine will take away stress, anger, and worry. The odor of jasmine from absolute is intensely floral, warm, rich and highly diffusive with a peculiar waxy-herbaceous, oily-fruity and tea-like undertone.

Juniper Oil (*junipers communis*): The juniper shrub grows wild all over central and southern Europe. Juniper oil, also called juniperberry oil, is obtained from the fresh or dried crushed berry or the fermented byproduct of beverage production in Europe. Both oils have a similar odor but differ in composition. Only the first method yields the true juniper oil which is a white or very pale yellow liquid. Juniper oil is a vasoconstrictor, is antiseptic, astringent, and antiinflammatory. It is especially well suited for cleansing the skin and for care of watery skin and in cellulitis preparations. It is used in facial masks and facial steam baths and leaves the skin tight and well cared for. Other applications are for treatment of acne, dandruff, and dermatitis. Juniper oil has a fresh, yet warm, rich-balsamic, woody-sweet and pine-needle-like odor.

Lavender Oil (*lavendula officinalis*): Lavender is a wild-growing or cultivated plant native to the Mediterranean countries. Lavender oil is steam distilled from freshly cut flower tops and stalks of the plant. It is a colorless or pale yellow liquid and contains linalyl, geranyl, geraniol, linalool, and cineol. Lavender is universally used in natural cosmetic preparations and is a valued medicinal oil. It is antibacterial, antiseptic, antifungal, anodyne. It is used for soothing of inflamed skin, and fosters regeneration of skin cells. It is useful for all skin types since it regulates sebum production. It is effective in treating acne, eczema, dermatitis, boils and burns. It has been shown as one of the most effective essential oils for natural cosmetic products and is also effective as an insecticide. The odor of lavender oil is sweet, floral-herbaceous refreshing with a pleasant, balsamic-woody undertone. An almost fruity-sweet top note is only of short duration.

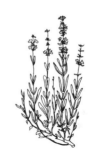

Fig. 61 *Lavender (lavendula officinalis)*

Lemon Oil (*citrus limomum*): The lemon tree is believed to be native to East India and Burma but is now cultivated all over the world and especially in California. This essential oil is expressed from the peels of ripe lemon. Lemon oil is a yellow to greenish-yellow mobile liquid. It contains mainly terpenes (pinene, limonene), and linalool, linalyl, and geranyl acetate. It is astringent, antibacterial, antiseptic, cleansing, and promotes cell regeneration (antiaging). It has been successfully applied to oily skin to reduce sebum production and to tighten the skin. Lemon oil is slightly bleaching and is used to treat freckles. It helps with brittle finger- and toe-nails, and is a proven remedy for chapped and rough skin. It is further used for blond hair care, helps with itching skin, dandruff, and healing of wounds. After treatment with lemon oil, or perfumes containing lemon oil, direct exposure to sunlight must be avoided since it increases the sensitivity of the skin to ultraviolet light and promotes tanning and sunburn.

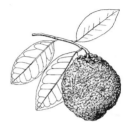

Fig. 62 *Lemon (citrus limomum)*

Lemongrass Oil (*cymbopogon flexuosus, citratus*): Both species are native to East India and Shrilanka but are now distributed all over the world. Lemongrass oil is steam distilled from the leaves (grass) of the plant. It is a yellow to amber colored liquid. Its main constituents are citral. Lemongrass oil is antibacterial, antiseptic, and is effective against fungal infections. It is used by the cosmetic industry as fragrance in soaps and in skin toners. It is an effective compound in natural insect repellants. Because some people are allergic to lemongrass oil, it is used in small amounts and not extensively in natural skin and hair care preparations. The odor is very peculiar, warm woody and yet fresh, grassy.

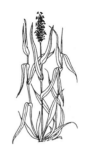

Fig. 63 *Lemongrass (cymbopogon flexuosus)*

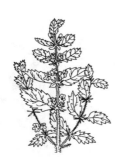

Fig. 64 *Melissa (melissa officinalis)*

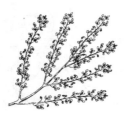

Fig. 65 *Myrrh (commiphora molmol)*

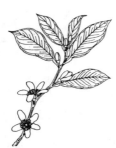

Fig. 66 *Neroli (citrus aurantium)*

Melissa Oil (*melissa officinalis*): Melissa is a small plant native to central and southern Europe and has been valued as a medicinal plant for thousands of years. The oil is distilled in very small amounts in Germany and France. This product has the reputation of being the most frequently adulterated oil in the industry. The essential oil sold as melissa oil is usually distilled with lemon oil, verbena oil, lemongrass oil and various mixtures and contains only a small fraction of the actual essential oil. Its composition is very similar to the cutting oils, mainly citral and citronella. Melissa oil has been definitely shown to have a calming effect and is used in calming and relaxing bath oils and foam baths.

Myrrh Oil (*commiphora molmol, abyssinica*): Both species of the tree are grown in various parts of eastern Africa and southern Arabia. Myrrh oil is obtained by steam distillation of crude myrrh oleo-gum-resin. It is a pale yellow to pale orange liquid whose composition has not been well analyzed. Egyptians used it for body care thousands of years ago. Myrrh oil is used in antiaging, antiwrinkle products and is said to promote new cell formation. It is antiinflammatory, antiseptic, antifungal, and astringent. It positively influences the healing process of skin suffering from dermatitis, wet eczema, or similar ailments.It is used as an ingredient in mouth washes to alleviate bad breath. The odor of myrrh oil is warm-spicy, with a peculiar sharp balsamic, slightly medicinal top note.

Neroli Oil (*citrus aurantium*): Neroli oil is distilled from the flowers of the cultivated bitter orange tree. It is a pale yellow oil which becomes darker and more viscous with aging. Its main constituents are geraniol, linalool, nerol, indol, and jasmon. Neroli oil promotes new cell generation, is antiinflammatory, and acts as an anodyne (painful skin). It is especially used for dry and aging skin. Its calming and aphrodisiac odor is valued as a bath oil or bath additive. Neroli oil has a very powerful light and refreshing floral top note but its tenacity is very poor.

Niaouli Oil (*melaleuca viridiflora*): The tree is native to Australia and one of several similar species that include the tea tree. The oil is produced by steam distillation from the leaves of the tree. It is a pale yellow to greenish-yellow liquid that contains mainly cineol, eucalyptol, and terpenes. Its application in natural cosmetics is mainly as a cleansing and healing compound. It is antibacterial, antiseptic, and used in acne preparations to treat inflammations of the skin, and sunburns. It also promotes the formation of new cells. Niaouli oil, has a strong, fresh, sweet-camphoraceous, but cooling, odor, reminiscent of eucalyptus oil.

Olibanum Oil (*boswellia carterii*): See Frankincense oil.

Orange Oil, Sweet (*citrus aurantium*): It is believed that the orange tree originated in the Far East in the Himalayas and southwestern China. Sweet orange oil is mainly produced in the United States either by steam distillation or cold expression from orange peels. The color is very pale yellow or almost colorless for the distilled oil and yellow to dark orange for the expressed oil. The main constituents are citral, citronellol, and limonene. When applied to the skin, orange oil is antibacterial, astringent, used for skin toning, treatment of acne, and for treatment of cellulitis. As with all citrus oils, direct exposure to sunlight after treatment with orange oil should be avoided since it increases the sensitivity of the skin to ultraviolet light and promotes tanning and sunburn. The odor of cold pressed orange oil is sweet, light and fresh, distinctly reminiscent of scratched sweet orange peel.

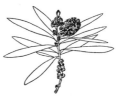

Fig. 67 *Niauli (melaleuca viridiflora)*

Patchouli Oil (*pogostemon cablin*): Patchouli is a small plant that originated in the Philippine Islands and Indonesia where most of the oil is still produced. Patchouli oil is produced by steam distillation from the leaves of the plant. It is a dark orange or brownish-colored liquid and contains mainly eugenol, patchoulol, and patchulene. Patchouli oil is antiinflammatory, antibacterial, antifungal, and supports generation of new cells. It is recommended for the care of acne, aging skin, chapped skin, and for dandruff conditions. The oil has an extremely rich, sweet, herbaceous, aromatic-spicy and woody-balsamic odor.

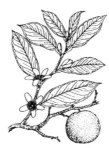

Fig. 68 *Orange (citrus aurantium)*

Peppermint Oil (*mentha piperita*): The peppermint plant is native to southern Europe. It is now cultivated in the United States, which is the largest producer of the oil. Peppermint oil is steam distilled from the partially dried herb and is a pale yellow or pale olive colored liquid. Its main constituents are menthol and limonene. Peppermint oil is used in natural cosmetics for skin cleansers because of its antiseptic, toning, and antiinflammatory properties. It is well suited for treatment of oily skin, acne, blackheads, and pimples. In addition, it is effective against itching skin, inflammations of the skin, and dandruff. The characteristic odor of peppermint oil is fresh, strong, somewhat grassy-minty with a deep balsamic-sweet undertone.

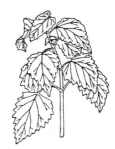

Fig. 69 *Patchouli (pogostemon cablin)*

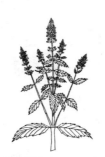

Fig. 70 *Peppermint (mentha piperita)*

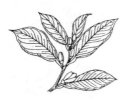

Fig. 71 *Petitgrain (citrus aurantium)*

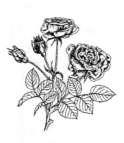

Fig. 72 *Rose (rosa damascena)*

Petitgrain Oil (*citrus aurantium*): Petitgrain oil is distilled from the leaves and twigs of the cultivated bitter orange tree. Its pale yellow to amber oil becomes darker and more viscous with aging. Its main constituents are geraniol, linalool, nerol, indol, andjasmon. Petitgrain oil promotes new cell generation, is antiinflammatory, and anodyne (for painful skin). It is especially used for dry and aging skin. Its calming and aphrodisiac odor is valued as a bath oil or bath additive. Petitgrain oil has a very powerful light and refreshing floral top note but its tenacity is very poor.

Rose Oil (*rosa damascena, otto, gallica, centifolia, alba*):
(The following properties of rose otto are representative of rose oils from other species.) Rose Otto is steam distilled from the flowers of rosa damascena and is a pale yellow, or slightly olive-yellow oil. The minimum perception of true rose oil for humans is one part in 25,000. It consists mainly of geraniol, citronellol, nerol, and eugenol. The benefits of rose oil in natural cosmetics and aromatherapy are numerous and is only limited by the high price of the oil (approximately $200 per ounce wholesale). It is astringent, toning, antiseptic, antiinflammatory, regenerative, and promotes the formation of new cells. It is used for general skin care and especially for dry, sensitive, and aging skin. It is effective as long-term treatment of fragile and broken capillaries. The odor of rose Otto is warm, deep floral, slightly spicy and immensely rich, truly reminiscent of red roses, often with nuances of honey.

Rosemary Oil (*rosmarinus officinalis*): This plant grows abundantly wild in Europe, Asia, and northern Africa. Rosemary oil is steam distilled from the flowers, leaves, and twigs of the plant. It is a pale yellow or almost colorless liquid and contains mainly borneol, lineol, camphene, and pinene. Rosemary oil has the reputation of helping prevent hair loss and strengthening thin hair. It has been used successfully to treat burns (sunburns), rheumatic complaints, muscle pain (massage oil), and eczema. It is astringent, antiseptic, and is used in cleansing creams and lotions and in skin toners. It improves skin metabolism and circulation and is used in hair shampoos and conditioners. Furthermore, it is a popular invigorating bath additive. The initial odor of rosemary oil is fresh, woody herbaceous, somewhat minty-forest-like. This note vanishes quickly and yields to a clean woody-balsamic, dry-herbaceous note that is quiet tenacious.

Rosewood Oil (*aniba roseodora*): The rosewood tree is a tropical, wild-growing evergreen tree from the Amazon basin. Rosewood oil, also known as Bois de Rose oil, is steam distilled from sawdust and chips of the rosewood lumber. It is a colorless or yellow-pale liquid and consist mainly of linalool. It is antibacterial and can be applied to all skin types to tone the skin and make it supple. It is used to strengthen connecting tissues, is a deodorant, and is also used for care of dark hair. Rosewood oil has a refreshing, sweet-woody, somewhat floral-spicy odor.

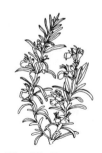

Fig. 73 *Rosemary (rosmarinus officinalis)*

Sage Oil (*salvia officinalis*): The sage bush is a wild-growing plant in several of the republics of the former Yugoslavia. Sage oil is distilled from the dried leaves of the plant. Dalmatian sage oil is a pale yellow liquid and consists mainly of borneol, salviol, cineol, and thujon. It is antiseptic, reduces perspiration, and stimulates blood circulation. It contains estrogen-like substances and is used to tighten the skin and in natural antiaging and antiwrinkle cosmetics and in preventive hair loss preparations. Sage oil is astringent and can heal dermatitis and eczema. It is used in invigorating bath preparations and to soothe rheumatic complaints. Sage oil has a strong, warm-spicy herbaceous and camphoraceous odor.

Sandalwood Oil (*santalum album*): The tree originates in India, Sri Lanka, Indonesia and surrounding islands. Sandalwood oil is steam distilled from the coarse powdered billets and roots of the tree. The oil is a viscous liquid with a pale yellow to yellow color, and is one of the oldest known fragrance materials. It is antiseptic, astringent, and promotes formation of new skin cells. It is a valuable skin care ingredient for all skin types and especially for inflamed, chapped, cracked, or fissured skin. It has been successfully used to control acne and itching skin. It gives hair a silky shine and is used in hair care products for dark hair. Sandalwood oil has a sweet-woody and almost animal-balsamic tenacious odor that remains uniform in time.

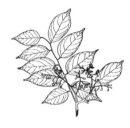

Fig. 74 *Rosewood (aniba roseodora)*

Tea Tree Oil (*melaleuca alternifolia*): The tea tree is one of the smaller melaleuca species and originates in Australia. Tea tree oil is steam distilled from the leaves of the tree. It is a pale yellowish-green or almost clear mobile liquid. This oil has served as an antiseptic for many years with a scientifically proven germ and fungus killing potency and high penetration power. In natural cosmetics tea tree oil is used to prevent and treat fungal infections (athlete's foot), inflammations of the nail bed, herpes, and forms of dermatitis. It is used in cleansing lotions for treatment of

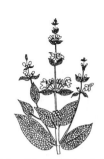

Fig. 75 *Sage (salvia officinalis)*

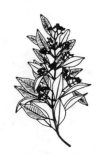

Fig. 76 *Sandalwood (sentalum album)*

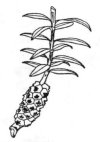

Fig. 77 *Tea tree (melaleuca alternifolia)*

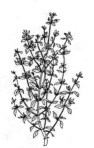

Fig. 79 *Thyme (thymus vulgaris)*

pimples. A comparative study of tea tree oil versus benzoyl peroxide (a synthetic chemical) in the treatment of acne showed comparable results but no side effects from using tea tree oil. The odor of tea tree oil is warm-spicy, aromatic-terpenic.

Thyme Oil (*thymus vulgaris*): Thyme oil is steam distilled from the partially-dried herb that abundantly grows wild in countries surrounding the Mediterranean Sea, North Africa, and in some former Russian republics. It is a brownish-red, orange-red or brown colored liquid. The main constituents are thymol, carvacrol, and terpene. Thyme oil is one of the most potent antiseptic essential oils. Only one part of thyme oil will kill all the bacteria in 1,000 parts of raw sewage. Its applications in natural cosmetics are manifold. It increases circulation, promotes metabolism and is used in healing preparations for oily skin and damaged skin. Thyme oil invigorates the scalp and is therefore found in hair shampoos, hair and scalp treatments, and preventative hair loss preparations. In bath preparations it is used to treat physical, nervous, and emotional exhaustion, and in massage oils as an ingredient to ease muscle pains, rheumatic complaints, and arthritis. The thyme oil fragrance is rich and powerful, sweet, and warm-herbaceous, somewhat spicy and distinctly aromatic.

Ylang Ylang Oil (*canangium odoratum*): The ylang ylang tree is native to Indonesia and the Philippines. The oil is produced by water distillation from the freshly picked flowers of the plant. It is a pale yellow oil that contains mainly eugenol, geraniol, linalool, saffron, and ylanol. It is used to normalize sebum production for all skin types, in preventive hair preparations, and to stimulate the scalp. It is frequently added to bath preparations and is said to have aphrodisiac properties. Ylang ylang oil has a very powerful, floral and intensively sweet odor.

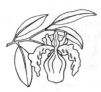

Fig. 78 *Ylang ylang (canagium odorata)*

Table 8 Essential Oils for Skin and Hair Care

Essential Oil	Properties
Benzoin balm (styrax benzoin)	antiinflammatory, antibacterial, deodorizing, calming, healing, improves skin elasticity; indications: cracked and chapped skin, dermatitis, dry skin, itching skin, skin irritation, skin rashes, wounds
Bergamot oil (citrus bergamia)	antibacterial, astringent, antiperspirant, deodorant, normalizes sebum production, healing; indications: acne, dandruff, eczema, herpes, oily skin seborrheic conditions
Cajaput oil (melaleuca leucadendron)	antibacterial, anodyne, antiinflammatory, expectorant; indications: acne, dandruff, hair loss, psoriasis
Caraway oil (carum carvi)	promotes generation of new tissue; indications: infected wounds, eczema
Cedarwood oil (cedrus virginiana)	antibacterial, antifungal, astringent, calming, deodorant; indications: dandruff, dermatitis, hair loss, itching skin, oily hair, seborrheic conditions
Chamomile oil (matricaria chamomilla, anthemis nobilis)	antiallergenic, antiinflammatory, antibacterial, astringent, healing, soothing, healing, vasoconstrictor; indications: acne, dermatitis, eczema, inflamed skin, sensitive skin, fragile capillaries
Cistus oil (cistus ladaniferus)	drying, wound healing; indications: ulcers, wounds
Clary Sage oil (salvia sclarea)	deodorant, estrogen-like ingredients, vitalizing; indications: dandruff, aging skin, hair loss
Coriander oil (coriandrum sativum)	analgesic; indications: rheumatic or muscular pain
Cypress oil (cupressus sempervirens)	astringent, deodorant, insect repellant, vasoconstrictor; indications: oily skin, perspiration (feet etc), varicose veins

Essential Oil	Properties
Eucalyptus oil (eucalyptus globulus)	antiinflammatory, antibacterial, estrogen-like ingredients, expectorant, insect repellant, promotes formation of new cells, rubefacient; indications: aging skin, infections, inflammations, herpes
Fennel oil (foeniculum vulgare)	astringent, antibacterial, antiinflammatory, antiwrinkle, cleanser, detoxifier; indications: aging skin, cellulitis, water retention, muscle tone
Fir oil (abies sibirica, alba)	antibacterial, deodorizing, expectorant, rubefacient, soothing, tonic; indications: asthma, respiratory weakness, rheumatic complaints, stress
Frankincense oil (boswellia carterii)	antiwrinkle, astringent, promotes new cell generation, revitalizing, tonic, vulnerary; indications: aged skin, dry and rough skin, inflammations
Geranium oil (pelargonium graveolens)	antibacterial, antiinflammatory, astringent, deodorizing, lymphatic stimulant, promotes new cell generation; indications: acne, aged skin, cellulitis, dermatitis, fungus, herpes, oily skin, seborrheic conditions
Ginger oil (zingiber officinale)	antibacterial, astringent; indications: infections, skin care
Hyssop oil (hysoppus officinalis)	expectorant, healing; indications: respiratory system, dermatitis, eczema, wounds and inflammations
Jasmine absolute (jasminum officinale)	antibacterial, antiinflammatory, aphrodisiac, moisturizing, healing, soothing; indications: dry skin, sensitive skin, dermatitis, stress
Juniper oil (juniperus communis)	astringent, antiinflammatory, antibacterial, cleanser, detoxifier, vasoconstrictor; indications: acne, aging skin, cellulitis, dandruff, dermatitis, eczema, watery skin
Lavender oil (lavendula officinalis)	antibacterial, anodyne, antifungal, antiinflammatory, insect repellant, promotes new cells generation, regulates sebum production, soothing; indications: acne, dermatitis, eczema, oily skin, sunburns

Essential Oil	Properties
Lemon oil (citrus limomum)	antibacterial, astringent, lymphatic stimulant, promotes new cells generation, regulates sebum production, tonic; <u>indications</u>: aging skin, brittle nails, chapped skin, freckles, dandruff, inflammations, itching skin,
Melissa oil (melissa officinalis)	antibacterial, insect repellant, healing; <u>indications</u>: acne, bruised skin, dermatitis, eczema, viral infections, calming
Lemon balm oil (melissa officinalis)	see Melissa oil
Lemongrass oil (cymbopogon flexuosus, citratus)	antibacterial, antifungal, astringent, deodorizer, insect repellant, tonic; <u>indications</u>: fungal infections, large pores
Lime oil (citrus aurantifolia)	see lemon oil
Myrrh oil (commiphora myrrha)	antiaging, antifungal, antiinflammatory, antiwrinkle, astringent, revitalizing, promotes formation of new cells, tonic, expectorant; <u>indications</u>: aged skin, catarrhal conditions, dermatitis, eczema, aging skin, dry skin
Neroli oil (citrus auranticum)	antiinflammatory, anodyne, aphrodisiac, calming, promotes new cell generation, soothing; <u>indications</u>: sensitive skin, dry skin, aging skin,
Niaouli oil (melaleuca viridiflora)	antibacterial, expectorant, healing, promotes new cell generation, stimulant; <u>indications</u>: acne, burn wounds, respiratory system, sinusitis
Nutmeg oil (myristica fragrans)	analgesic, antibacterial; <u>indications</u>: muscular pain
Orange oil, sweet (citrus aurantium)	antibacterial, astringent, toning; <u>indications</u>: acne, cellulitis, skin care
Palmarosa oil (cymbopogon martini)	antibacterial, moisturizing, promotes new cell generation, soothing stimulant; <u>indications</u>: acne, dermatitis, skin care, dry skin

Essential Oil	Properties
Patchouli oil (pogostemon patchouli)	antiinflammatory, antifungal, antiwrinkle, promotes formation of new cells; <u>indications</u>: acne, aged skin, cracked and chapped skin, dandruff, dermatitis, eczema, fungal infections
Peppermint oil (mentha piperita)	antiinflammatory, cleanser, decongestant, anodyne; <u>indications</u>: acne, blackheads, pimples, dandruff, dermatitis, itching skin, muscular pain, oily skin
Pine oil (pinus sylvetris)	antibacterial, deodorizing, expectorant, rubefacient, soothing, tonic; <u>indications</u>: asthma, respiratory weakness, rheumatic complaints, stress
Rose oil (rose damascena, rose centifolia)	astringent, healing, moisturizing, promotes formation of new cells; <u>indications</u>: aged skin, eczema, fragile and broken capillaries, sensitive skin, dry skin
Rosemary oil (rosemarinus officinalis)	antibacterial, astringent, circulatory stimulant, regulates sebum discharge, scalp stimulant; <u>indications</u>: acne, dermatitis, eczema, dry skin, aged skin, antiwrinkle, dandruff, hair loss, oily hair, sunburns, rheumatic complaints
Rosewood oil (Aniba roseodora)	antibacterial, deodorant, hair conditioner, tonic; <u>indications</u>: aging skin, dark hair care, strengthens weak connecting skin tissues
Sage oil (salvia officinalis)	antiaging, antiperspirant, antibacterial, astringent, healing, regulator of sebum production, soothing; <u>indications</u>, acne, dermatitis, eczema, dandruff, dermatitis, eczema, excessive sweating, hair loss, rheumatic complaints
Sandalwood oil (santalum album)	antibacterial, antiinflammatory, astringent, hair conditioner, healing, moisturizing, promotes formation of new skin cells, soothing; <u>indications</u>: acne, cracked, chapped skin, dry skin, itching skin, dark hair care
Spearmint oil (mentha spicata)	cleanser, decongestant, analgesic; <u>indications</u>: acne, dermatitis, muscular pain
Spruce oil (picea alba)	antibacterial, deodorizing, expectorant, rubefacient, soothing, tonic; <u>indications</u>: asthma, respiratory weakness, rheumatic complaints, stress

Essential Oil	Properties
Tea tree oil (melaleuca alternifolia)	antibacterial, antifungal, expectorant; indications: abscesses, acne, athlete's foot, dandruff, hair care, hair loss, herpes, inflamed nail beds, pimples, oily skin, respiratory problems, skin irritation, skin rashes
Thyme oil (thymus vulgaris)	antibacterial, antifungal, aphrodisiac, circulatory stimulant, healing, normalizes sebum production, scalp stimulant; indications: hair loss, dermatitis, eczema, damaged skin, oily skin, rheumatic complaints, stress, muscle pain
Vetiver oil (vetiveria zizanoides)	rubefacient; indications: muscular pain, arthritis
Ylang ylang oil (canagum odoratum)	aphrodisiac, normalizes sebum production, scalp stimulant; indications: oily skin, hair growth, frigidity

Vitamins

Vitamins are organic substances that occur in living things in minute quantities. They are vital for proper growth and maintenance of health in plants and animals. Green leaves are the laboratories in which plant vitamins are manufactured. Seeds and fruits also contain vitamins which plants provide to nourish the next generation. Animals obtain their vitamins from plants or from animals who eat plants. Some animals can manufacture several vitamins they need in their own body. Fifteen vitamins have been recognized and analyzed to date. Scientists believe that many more probably exist and are equally essential for health.

The discovery of vitamins is an exciting story. For centuries people suffered from diseases (caused by vitamin deficiencies) that at the time could not be explained or cured. At the beginning of this century, scientists suspected for the first time that there may be more in foodstuffs than fats, proteins, carbohydrates, and minerals. It was found that laboratory animals were still dying from malnutrition although all the above substances were present in their diets. Further research identified substances that are active in very minute quantities which can prevent diseases like beriberi, pellagra, pernicious anemia, scurvy, rickets, and many others.

Vitamins are normally ingested and enter the blood stream through the intestines. They are distributed throughout the body with every cell removing its share of these vital substances from the capillary network. The skin (at the periphery of the human body) is the last to be supplied, capturing whatever nutrients and vitamins are left over. Therefore, the skin is notoriously sensitive to vitamin deficiencies because the circulation does not supply it with copious amounts of nutrition. Poor circulation aggravates this condition considerably. The first indications of vitamin deficiencies are usually found in the skin.[12] A few examples of skin ailments which can be directly attributed to vitamin deficiencies are presented in Table 9.

Table 9 Signs of Vitamin Deficiencies

Clinical Deficiency Signs	Vitamin
Infection and ulceration of the eye; scaling and dryness or the eyelids; hard, dry, and itching skin	Vitamin A
Itching burning eyes; lesions in the corner of the mouth and inflammation of the tongue	Vitamin B2 (riboflavin)
Itching inflammation of skin exposed to sunlight; rough and dry skin (symptoms of pellagra)	Vitamin B3 (niacin)
Eczema-like outbreak on face and body; skin and mouth lesions	Vitamin B6 (pyridoxine)
Seborrheic dermatitis and peeling skin dermatitis	Biotin
Skin lesions, bruises, bleeding gums, and loose teeth (symptoms of scurvy)	Vitamin C

Modern research has shown that the skin can be readily penetrated by certain substances, including vitamins. Therefore, it makes good sense to supply vitamins to the skin topically by means of creams and lotions. Many cosmetic manufacturers have started to include vitamins in their products. Technically speaking, the FDA may consider such cosmetics as drugs, misbranded drugs, or misbranded cosmetics if the label declaration is supplemented with statements implying prevention, treatment of disease, or able to affect the structure or function of the skin, because vitamins can dramatically effect the structure and function of the skin.

It is beyond the ability of the layman and difficult for physicians to diagnose symptoms of skin problems (like erythema, dermatitis, or seborrhea) that are caused by marginal vitamin deficiencies. Through some study and observations of your own, you can spot potential deficiencies and find a remedy for certain skin conditions. Vitamin deficiencies do not

---

[12]   Miller S.J., Nutritional deficiency and the skin, Division of Dermatology, University of California, San Diego School of Medicine, *J. Am. Acad. Dermatol.*, 1989 Jul, 21(1), 1-30.

happen overnight. Long-term marginal deficiencies coupled with stress, disease, and poor nutrition can manifest outright deficiencies on the skin. The elderly are especially susceptible to these conditions. In our modern diet we consume substances from which almost all vitamins have been removed (sugar, white flour, rice, and processed oils). We can no longer be sure that sufficient quantities of vitamins are supplied to the skin through food intake. I recommend that you supplement these vital substances topically to your skin. This can also serve to combat against the effects of atmospheric pollutants on the skin.

The following is a short description of vitamins and their beneficial effects on human skin and hair. A summary of vitamins used for skin and hair care is provided in Table 10.

Ascorbic acid : see Vitamin C

Biotin: Biotin is part of the Vitamin B complex and is a sulfur-containing organic compound. It occurs naturally in minute amounts in a number of foods (liver .0001 %) and is also synthesized in the lower gastrointestinal tract by microorganisms. It is a coenzyme and an integral part of the enzyme system in human tissues and necessary for the metabolism of carbohydrates, proteins and fats, especially of unsaturated fatty acids. It is most plentiful in yeast, liver, eggs, and in a variety of fish and grains. The vitamin is needed for maintenance of skin, hair, and sebaceous glands. Low activity of biotin enzymes can be produced by high intake of proteins including raw egg white. Biotin deficiencies result in a variety of symptoms including skin rashes and hair loss in humans which can usually be reversed by supplying adequate amounts of biotin.[13] Biotin is expensive and not usually found in all multi-vitamin preparations. It is stable and water soluble and can be applied topically to skin and scalp through creams and lotions to ensure adequate supply.

Carotene: also see Retinol: Carotene is a generic name for a number of substances that are converted in the liver to Vitamin A. The most important one is β-carotene which occurs in carrots, spinach and other green leafy vegetables. It has been determined that six parts of β-carotene is equivalent to one part of retinol. β-Carotene is receiving great attention as an inhibitor of a variety of cancers in humans, including skin cancer.[14]

Niacin (Vitamin B3): The term niacin is used in a generic sense for both nicotinic acid and nicotinamide. Nicotinic acid and nicotinamide are both stable and water soluble. Nicotinic

---

[13] Mock D.M., Skin manifestations of biotin deficiency, Department of Pediatrics, University of Iowa Hospitals and Clinics, Iowa City, *Semin. Dermatol.*, 1991 Dec, 10(4), 296-302.

[14] Malone W.F., Studies evaluating antioxidants and beta-carotene as chemopreventives, Chemoprevention Branch, National Cancer Institute, Bethesda, MD, *Am. J. Clin. Nutr.*, 1991 Jan, 53(1 Suppl), 305S-313S.

acid is found in small amounts in liver, yeast, milk, alfalfa, and legumes but is mostly produced synthetically. Both forms of niacin perform the same function but have different pharmacological properties. The body converts both compounds into a number of coenzymes that are necessary for both cellular and systemic metabolism. Common foods that are rich in niacin include liver, heart, and kidneys of beef, turkey, chicken, sunflower seeds, whole wheat flour, and yeast. There are still many regions on this planet where the population suffers from pellagra, a niacin deficiency that causes dermatitis, inflammation of the mucous membranes, and dementia. In a nationwide survey conducted by the U.S. Department of Health, Education, and Welfare, called the First Health and Nutritional Examination Survey (HANES), it was found that many Americans showed clinical signs of niacin deficiency, mainly women and the elderly, because of poor dietary habits, regardless of income. Nicotinic acid is a vasodilator (expands blood vessels) and is used in preventive hair loss preparations to increase circulation of the skin and scalp and to promote skin metabolism.

PABA (p-aminobenzoic acid): PABA is one of the lesser known constituents of the Vitamin B complex and is widely distributed in nature (yeast). It is one of the basic constituents of the folic acid vitamin, is involved with the utilization of pantothenic acid, and also is a coenzyme needed for the metabolism of proteins and the production of blood cells. PABA has been shown to be a very effective sunscreen by a Harvard team of researchers. Follow-on studies confirmed that PABA and its esters gave superior protection on both lip and skin when compared with all other sun screen agents. Unfortunately, p-aminobenzoic acid by itself causes photosensitivity and dermatitis in some people (Ref. 120). Esters of PABA, like octyl dimethyl PABA, also called Padimate O, have shown little adverse effects so far and are part of many sunscreen preparations.

Pantothenic acid: The name of pantothenic acid is derived from the Greek name pantos, meaning everywhere, since it occurs in all living cells. It is a B-complex vitamin and takes part in carbohydrate metabolism and synthesis of such vital compounds as sterols, steroid hormones, and others. Deficiencies of pantothenic acid in animal diets cause a variety of adverse growth effects, including abnormalities of skin, hair, and feathers. Although no such symptoms have been observed in humans, the cosmetic industry uses pantothenic acid and its derivatives (panthenol, dexpanthenol, etc.) extensively as hair conditioning agents.

Pyridoxine (Vitamin B6): Pyridoxine is a water soluble vitamin and plays an important role in the maintenance of healthy skin, and is necessary for the breakdown and metabolism of carbohydrates, fats, and the formation of blood and antibodies. Good dietary sources of pyridoxine include meat, whole grains, wheat germs, and dried beans. Pyridoxine deficiencies include skin disorders, like dermatitis, cracked lips, inflammation of the mouth and tongue. These deficiencies can be caused by taking estrogen, by malabsorption disorders in humans, and alcoholism. Research shows that a large sector of the U.S. population may suffer from Vitamin B6 deficiencies because of poor dietary habits (processed foods contain less pyridoxine), and because of high protein consumption.

B. Leonard Snyder, M.D., reported in Obstetrical and Gynecological News, (May 1, 1974), that he gave daily Vitamin B6 (Pyridoxine) supplements to teenagers whose acne was under control except for flare-ups just prior to menstruation. Seventy-five percent of the girls reduced their acne flare-up substantially as a result of this treatment. Other doctors have reported success using Vitamin B6 in treating a skin disease called seborrhea. Vitamin B6 is not generally used in cosmetic products except for specialty creams and lotions.

Retinoids: Synthetic Vitamin A derivatives, called retinoids, have been used to treat a number of clinical skin conditions, including cystic acne and various forms of ichthyosis, and psoriasis. Because of the toxicity of existing retinoids, newer Vitamin A derivatives are being developed and continue to be evaluated. Because of their toxicity, synthetic retinoids must only be used under a doctor's care and should not be used in cosmetic products.

Retinol (Vitamin A): Retinol, also called the growth vitamin, is an alcohol-like organic compound that occurs bound to a fatty acid in some animals (retinol esters) like fish liver oils, organ meats (liver), butter, and eggs. It is insoluble in water but dissolves readily in oils. It is frequently marketed as Vitamin A palmitate, dissolved in plant oils, which is stable and is readily absorbed by the skin and converted in the body into Vitamin A. Many plants and animals also produce carotene, a precursor Vitamin A compound that is converted into Vitamin A in the body.

Vitamin A plays an important role in RNA synthesis which produce new and healthy cells in skin and body. The epidermis of your skin is especially sensitive to Vitamin A deficiencies since its basal layer continually generates new cells that keratinize and become the horny layer, the protective barrier of the body against the outside world. As a result of deficiencies, these cell prematurely die, harden, and plug the oil sacs and pores that give the skin a look that resembles goose pimples.

University of Pennsylvania researchers discovered that in most cases topically applied Vitamin A begins to clear up acne from three to five weeks after the initial treatment and returns the skin to normal usually within six months. Dermatologists at their annual meeting in Chicago in 1971 were so impressed by the results, they awarded the Pennsylvania researchers a silver medal for Research in Skin Disease. Further research by different teams largely confirmed the earlier result and additionally found that Vitamin A, when applied to the skin at an early stage, may prevent the formation of acne altogether. Vitamin A and its derivatives also have shown beneficial effects in controlling psoriasis, neoplastic processes, and most recently, reversal in extrinsically aged skin.[15] It has also been shown to be effective in preventing malignant skin cancer when applied early.[16] It also strengthens the immune

---

[15]   Boyd A.S., An overview of the retinoids, Department of Dermatology, School of Medicine, Texas Tech University Health Sciences Center, Lubbock 79430, *Am. J. Med.*, 1989 May, 86(5), 568-74.

[16]   Maugh, Thomas H., Vitamin A: a potential Protection from Carcinogens, *Science*, 27 December 1974.

system of the body and has shown to be effective in suppressing warts and hyper keratosis. Vitamin A is easily destroyed by a number of environmental conditions and compounds that occur as a result of pollution. Ultraviolet light, oxygen in the atmosphere, and nitrogen compounds (fertilizers present in all commercially grown vegetables, fruits and meats) readily destroy the vitamin. Meat preservatives (nitrites) also destroy Vitamin A and β-carotene as well. Since the skin is exposed to environmental pollution and carcinogens it makes great sense to supply this important vitamin topically using creams and lotions to avoid local deficiencies. Medical studies indicate that Vitamin A is effective in slowing down skin aging. In a randomized study with human subjects, results demonstrated a reduction in the number and depth of the wrinkles and a regression of the pigmented spots.[17]

Riboflavine (Vitamin B2): Riboflavine is an essential vitamin and plays an important role in cell metabolism. New tissue cannot be formed nor can damaged tissue be repaired unless this vitamin is available. Riboflavin deficiency in humans is characterized by growth failure in children, nerve degradation (particularly of the eyes), sore throat, seborrheic dermatitis of the face and extremities, and anemia. It is believed that an increasing sector of the population suffers from marginal deficiencies because of poor dietary habits and the consumption of highly processed foods (potato chips, crackers, cookies, doughnuts, ice creams, candies, and "instant" products) which contain little or no Vitamin B2. Riboflavine is easily destroyed by heat, alkali, ultraviolet radiation (i.e. when milk is irradiated to form Vitamin D), oral contraceptives, and alcohol. It is added to some skin lotions to ensure an ample supply to regenerate damaged skin due to UV radiation and pollution, and to promote the formation of healthy skin tissues overall. It has a strong orange color which gives cosmetic preparations a pinkish hue.

Tocopherol: see Vitamin E

Vitamin A: see Retinol

Vitamin B2: see Riboflavine

Vitamin B3: see Niacin

Vitamin B6: see Pyridoxine

Vitamin C (Ascorbic acid): This vitamin is widely distributed in the plant and animal kingdom and occurs in appreciable amounts in citrus fruits, hip berries and acerola. Most

---

[17]   Salagnac V., Leonard F., de-Lacharriere O., Le-Corre Y., Kalis-B, Traitement du vieillissement actinique par la vitamine A acide topique a differentes concentrations [Treatment of actinic aging with topical vitamin A acid in different concentrations], Service de Dermatologie, Hopital Sebastopol, Reims, *Rev. Fr. Gynecol. Obstet.*, 1991 Jun, 86(6), 458-60.

Vitamin C for human consumption today is manufactured synthetically. It is believed that because of a genetic deficiency man alone is unable to synthesize ascorbic acid and depends on external sources for sufficient amounts of Vitamin C. The vitamin plays an essential role in the activities of enzymes in human tissues and is important for the growth and maintenance of healthy bones and skin tissues. It strengthens the immune system and assists in healing wounds. Vitamin C is a natural antioxidant and a scavenger of free radicals similar to Vitamin E. Free radicals result from peroxidation of fatty acids that destroy the membranes of cells or alter the cell structure inside the body. The most convincing evidence for the involvement of Vitamin C in cancer prevention is the ability of ascorbic acid to prevent formation of nitrosamine and other N-nitroso compounds. In addition vitamin C supplementation was shown to inhibit skin cancer.[18] Animal tests have shown that the formation of cancer-causing cholesterol-∝-oxide in the skin by UV radiation was drastically reduced when high levels of Vitamin C were maintained in the skin.

Healthy collagen and elastin tissues in your skin minimize wrinkles and keeps it looking young. Vitamin C is indispensable for the formation of healthy collagen and it has been shown that the synthesis of collagen is significantly depressed in cases of ascorbic acid deficiency. Herpes zoster (shingles) is an infection of the nerves and causes a painful skin rash of small, crusting blisters. Doctors have reported that large doses of ascorbic acid can give prompt relief to the symptoms and pain, believed to be due to detoxification properties of Vitamin C.

Vitamin D: Vitamin D is a collective term for a number of related substances that include calciferol (Vitamin D2) and cholecalciferol (Vitamin D3). The richest source of dietary Vitamin D is fortified milk, oily fish, and dairy products. The skin can synthesize Vitamin D when exposed to sunlight. Very recently it was discovered that Vitamin D and its analogues have hormone-like functions and its derivatives are effective in treating certain skin disorders, like psoriasis.[19]

Vitamin E (tocopherol): Vitamin E is the collective term for similar substances of which α-tocopherol is the most prominent. These substances are found largely in plant materials, especially plant oils, alfalfa and lettuce. They are practically insoluble in water but freely soluble in oils. Vitamin E is essential for maintaining the activities of enzymes in the cells and for the formation of red blood cells. It protects lung and skin tissues from damage by pollutants and is a powerful free radical scavenger. There is convincing evidence for the involvement of Vitamin E in cancer prevention by inhibiting the formation of cancer-causing

---

[18]   Bird D.F., Update on the effects of vitamins A, C, and E and selenium on carcinogenesis. Source (Bibliographic citation), *Proc. Soc. Exp. Biol. Med.*, 1986 Dec, 183(3), 311-20.

[19]   Lowe K.E., Norman A.W., Vitamin D and psoriasis, Department of Biochemistry, University of California, Riverside CA, *Nutr. Rev.*, 1992 May, 50(5), 138-42.

nitrosamines and other n-nitroso compounds. In addition, Vitamin E was shown to inhibit skin cancer by itself.[20]

In the section on preservatives, the important role of vitamin E in reducing the formation of free radicals inside the body was emphasized. Premature aging of the body (and especially the skin) has been linked in several studies to unsaturated free fatty acid radicals and reactive oxygen- forming toxic peroxides that damage and permanently destroy cells. Polyunsaturated oils are much more prone to form free radicals in the body than are other oils. Consumption of polyunsaturated oils in our diet increases the need for additional Vitamin E.

Researchers at the Lawrence Berkeley Laboratory in California reported that Vitamin E can more than double the life of a human cell in an artificial test-tube environment. These cells usually reproduce about 50 times before dying. When they added Vitamin E to the cultured medium at about ten times the level normally observed in human tissue they found that the cell reproduced through 120 generations. Vitamin E, therefore, can become a dynamic weapon against premature aging and to combat wrinkles. It also promulgates the healing of burned skin without forming scars that are tender or contract. In addition, Vitamin E linoleate is a proven deep moisturizer that softens and tones dry lines of the skin. Every skin care preparation can benefit by including this versatile and valuable group of vitamins.

Table 10 Vitamins for Skin and Hair Care

Vitamin	Properties
Ascorbic Acid	see Vitamin C
B2 (riboflavin)	essential for formation of new healthy tissues; positive influence on healing sunburned skin; prevents pink eye (conjunctivitis), lip and mouth skin cracks
B3 (niacin)	nicotinic acid is a vasodilator; increases peripheral circulation; prevents and heals skin rashes; useful in hair loss preparations and scalp treatments
B6 (pyridoxine)	essential for DNA/RNA synthesis; prevents seborrheic and acne disorders as well as skin lesions
Biotin	essential for maintenance of skin (sebaceous glands) and hair; prevents seborrheic dermatitis and scaling of skin

[20]   Bird D.F., Update on the effects of vitamins A, C, and E and selenium on carcinogenesis. Source (Bibliographic citation), *Proc. Soc. Exp. Biol. Med.*, 1986 Dec, 183(3), 311-20

Vitamin	Properties
Carotene (vitamin A precursor, plant)	essential for cell synthesis; anticarcinogen; antioxidant; retards development of hardened skin cells, keeps cells younger
PABA (para-aminobenzoic acid)	sunscreen (Padimate O); prevents sunburn and possible prevention of skin cancer
pantothenic acid (vitamin B group)	moisturizing; can restore hair growth; strengthens hair follicles
Retinol	shown to reduce wrinkles and pigmented spot on the skin; prevents hard, dry, itching skin; infection and dryness of eyelids; normalizes dry skin and helps reversing damage due to UV radiation; protection of skin against carcinogens; successful treatment of warts and psoriasis
Vitamin E linoleate	prolongs life of human cells; moisturizer; antioxidant; see Vitamin E
Vitamin E acetate	penetrates deep into skin and helps protect against uv radiation and ozone exposure damage; antioxidant; see Vitamin E
Vitamin E (n-tocopherol)	prolongs life of human cells; neutralizes free radicals; antioxidant; inhibits skin cancer; heals skin ailments like eczema and ulcers,
Vitamin A	see Retinol
Vitamin D	shown to be effective in treating psoriasis and other skin disorders
Vitamin C (ascorbic acid), water soluble	essential for protein synthesis; blocks carcinogens; indispensable for collagen formation; antiwrinkle effect
Vitamin C palmitate (ascorbyl palmitate), oil soluble	essential for protein synthesis; blocks carcinogens; free radical scavenger; indispensable for connecting tissue formation; antiwrinkle effect

Chapter 4

Skin Care

Every person wants smooth, tight and supple skin. Skin tells a lot about its wearer because it is closely connected with the total circulatory system of the body. Skin provides indications of age, care, and habits. It is no surprise that many deficiencies inside the body first manifest themselves at the skin level. Internal ailments and improper nutrition also affect the skin. Skilled dermatologists can diagnose many external (caused by environmental influences) and internal (systemic) ailments by observing the skin. Misuse of alcohol, frequent use of tobacco, and environmental exposure also leave their mark. A deeply suntanned skin may demonstrate activity and health; unfortunately, it also signifies accelerated wrinkle formation and in extreme cases skin diseases and cancer.

Function of Skin

The skin consists of three parts: the subcutaneous layer, dermis, and epidermis (see Figure 80). The subcutaneous layer consists of loosely bound connective tissues with embedded pads of fat. These pads absorb pressure and blows from the outside and also serve as heat insulation. Fat also serves as an energy reserve for skin nourishment.

The dermis is also comprised of connective tissues, but these are much more tightly bound than in the subcutaneous layer. Its great strength and elasticity is attributed to the presence of collagen fiber bundles and the elastic net made of elastin. The dermis is penetrated by many capillary blood vessels. This is necessary for passing nutrients to the skin and for temperature regulation. Also necessary for temperature regulation are sweat glands,embedded in the dermis, which end in small pores leading outside the body. Finally, the \dermis contains hair roots and sebaceous glands (oil glands) that supply the necessary lubrication and make the skin and hair flexible. At the end of each hair bulb is a small muscle (the erector muscle) that causes this secretion to take place. After sustained exposure to cold temperature these muscles contract, causing the hair to stand up (since hair standing up provides better insulation). The result is what we commonly call goose pimples. This reaction

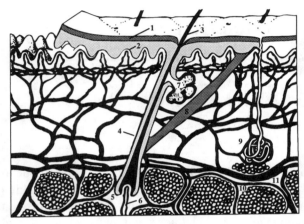

1. Horny layer.
2. Germinating layer.
3. Hair.
4. Follicle.
5. Hair bulb.
6. Capillaries.
7. Sebaceous gland.
8. Erector muscle.
9. Sweat gland.
10. Fatty tissues.
11. Blood vessels.

Fig. 80 *Cross section of skin*

is controlled by the pituitary gland and is a remnant from an earlier evolutionary period when the human body was covered with hair.

Above the dermis is the protective layer called the epidermis that divides into the germinating (basal) layer and horny layer respectively. In the germinating layer new cells are created continuously. The skin pigment, melanin, is formed by special cells called melanocytes whose activity is controlled by the pituitary gland in the brain. Exposure to sunlight increases the production of melanin, which protects the skin against the harmful effects of ultraviolet rays, darkening the skin in the process. Localized overproduction of melanin can cause pigmented spots called freckles.

After staying inside the epidermis for a period of time the cells move toward the outside, absorbing a horny substance called keratin. This causes the cells to stop their metabolic activity and form the horny layer. The main task of this layer (that is normally about 0.001 inches or about 20 cells thick) is to protect the deeper-lying skin from surface damage by mechanical or chemical means. The uppermost cells of the horny layer continuously form tiny scales that can detach themselves. In this fashion the entire epidermis renews itself completely about every 28 days. The most important functions of the skin are briefly described in the following paragraphs:

Respiratory Function: Besides forming a protective mantle for the body, the skin is also a respiratory organ. It absorbs oxygen from the air and performs about 2 percent of the total respiration of the body. Also, it secretes oil, sweat, and dross. The body normally loses about one quart of liquid per day through the skin. Two-thirds of this quantity is sweat and the rest is water.

Temperature Control Function: Additional water is lost to cool the body if the outside temperature is high, since evaporating water lowers the temperature of the body surface. In addition the skin becomes reddish (a sign of expanding blood vessels) which aids the heat flow and prevents overheating. When the outside temperature is cold, the blood vessels contract and the oil glands increase secretion. The skin becomes paler and goose pimples appear, preserving heat in the process. The skin, therefore, has the important function of regulating the heat budget of the body.

Hydrolipid Mantle: Two additional functions of the skin are to prevent too much moisture loss and over-hydration. The skin accomplishes these functions through the secretion of specific chemicals that form a special natural skin cream. These substances are fats that occur in living organisms in both the animal and plant world, and phospholipids and cholesterol that have emulsifying properties. The fats form a water soluble emulsion with phospholipids and cholesterol that can be penetrated by sweat. An oil film alone would prevent this from happening and would therefore interfere with the other vital functions of the skin such as preventing over-hydration. The hydrolipid mantle can be easily destroyed by using the wrong kind of soap or detergent. It takes the skin five to eight hours to restore this mantle on its own.

Acid Mantle: The acid mantle is another protective film formed by the skin. Its function is to suppress bacteria growth on the surface. Before treating this subject in any detail, an explanation is necessary about the pH value, which is a measure of the acidity or alkalinity in a liquid. The values of the pH scale range from zero to fourteen and are defined as the inverse logarithm of the hydrogen ion concentration. The neutral point is pure distilled water (which has the pH value of seven). The addition of acid lowers the pH value. Lemon juice, for instance, has a pH of about two. When an alkaline solution, like ammonia, is added to a solution, the pH increases. When an acid is added to a solution, the pH decreases (see Figure 81).

The acid mantle on the surface of the human skin normally has a pH between five and six and is therefore slightly acidic. The purpose of this film is to inhibit the growth of bacterial and other microorganisms. Cosmetic creams are usually adjusted to a pH value between five and six to match the actual skin acidity. The acid mantle is formed from the secretion of oil glands, sweat glands, and expelled carbon dioxide. The other function of this film is to act as a buffer system to prevent the shift of the pH value of the skin into the alkaline region when exposed to a limited amount of alkaline material. The buffer system

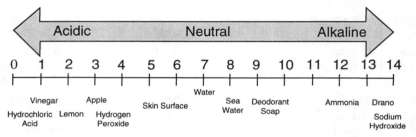

Fig. 81 *pH scale*

cannot neutralize the amount of alkali that is contained in regular soap or most detergents. As a result, the acid mantle is temporarily destroyed and the pH of the skin is temporarily increased. Although the acidity to the skin surface will be restored in a few hours, the exposure of the skin to substances with a pH value of eight or higher should be minimized. A high pH value of the skin makes the skin vulnerable because of increased bacterial growth and penetration, since alkaline substances also remove the oil barrier. Dry skin is especially sensitive to substances with higher pH values. Cleansing substances that are almost neutral are preferred and have been discussed in the section on gentle cleansing.

Composition of the Skin

The skin consists of proteins which are also the chief constituents of animal and plant bodies. Protein synthesis takes place in a living cell and is accomplished by the genetic materials called DNA (deoxyribonucleic acid) and RNA (ribonucleic acid). Cells form each type of protein from smaller building blocks (called amino acids) that are tailored for a specific function in the body. The main components of the skin and hair are fiber proteins that usually form fiber bundles. The most important groups of fiber proteins are collagen and elastin. Keratins are part of dead cells that form the protective top layer of skin and also occur in hair and fingernails.

Collagen

Collagen is the principal constituent of connecting tissues in humans and higher animals and can make up to one-third of the total weight of the body. Collagen molecules are very long and string-like. The molecular weight of these proteins is about 300,000 which corresponds to more than 50,000 atoms bonded together in a string forming a fibrous molecule. The fiber itself is made up of horizontal fibrils. The arrangement of these fibrils differs depending on the task they have to fulfill within the body. For example, collagen in the sinews forms fibrous bundles that are very strong but are not very elastic. To provide elasticity in the skin tissues, collagen fibers form a net-like structure (See Figure 82). Collagen has the ability to bind a great deal of water, which is an important attribute of

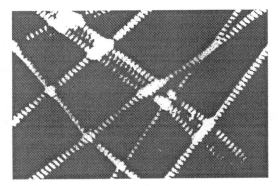

Fig. 82   *Collagen fibers under the microscope*

healthy skin. About 20 to 40 percent of all the water in the body is found in the skin. This is one reason why youthful skin looks so full, fresh, and smooth. With increasing age the soluble collagen transforms itself into insoluble collagen, which has a reduced ability to bind water causing the skin to become slack and form wrinkles. Skin with many wrinkles is also very dry skin. Collagen can also easily be damaged by light, especially ultraviolet (UV) rays. Therefore, skin exposed to UV radiation ages faster. The skin on the face, neck, and hands is normally exposed to this kind of radiation much more frequently than the rest of the body and correspondingly ages and loses its elasticity faster.

Elastin

While collagen has the more supportive and structural function in the skin, elastin forms a very elastic and stretchable net of connective tissue that is mainly responsible for the elasticity of the skin. Only one to two percent of the dry weight of skin consists of elastin.

With increasing age, fatty tissues attach themselves to the elastin fibers and prevent them from functioning properly. There is a simple test of elasticity you can perform on your skin. Pull up some skin from the back of your hand or face with the tips of two fingers and let go. The faster it returns to its initial shape the more elastic the skin is. If you try this with sunburned skin you will be amazed how much elasticity the skin has lost in the tanning process.

There are many cosmetic preparations on the market that freely use the names collagen and elastin trying to make you believe that these preparations can restore the lost elasticity of your skin and rebuild aging skin structure. As good as it sounds, this is impossible. The collagen and elastin molecules in those preparations are derived from animals and fortunately cannot penetrate the skin. If they could get into the cell structure of the skin, they would immediately be rejected by the body and attacked by the immune system. The only role they have in cosmetics is their ability to bind water and thus form a moist layer outside the skin.

Skin Permeability

Human skin is highly permeable to a large class of both beneficial and toxic materials. Medical research has established to what degree different substances can penetrate the skin. The findings show that significant amounts of cosmetic ingredients, including mutagenic and carcinogenic substances, penetrate the skin and end up in the blood stream. Still, many companies in the cosmetic industry choose ingredients for cosmetics based on the mistaken belief that the skin is a near perfect-barrier to the chemicals that are contained in cosmetic preparations. This belief went unchallenged until the 1960s when the much heralded but un-marketed miracle drug DMSO (Methyl Sulfoxide, RTECS # 48652) proved its ability to carry substances through the skin and into the body's tissues and blood stream. Today we know that all chemicals penetrate the skin to some degree and many do so in significant amounts. Modern medicine makes increasing use of this fact by delivering drugs transdermally. Medications to prevent sea sickness, chest pains (nitroglycerin), and hormonal deficiencies can today be placed in an adhesive patch for delivery through the skin.

The long-term effect on the body of daily application of dangerous and often toxic cosmetic ingredients, even when used in small amounts, has not been established. Since most consumers and cosmetic companies are only concerned with immediate allergic reactions and skin irritations, there has been little research into long-term adverse effects on the entire bodily system. To restore a particular function of the body, you may take drugs that cause side effects. These side effects may be worth enduring if the treatment is able to repair or maintain your health. The psychological benefits from the use of cosmetics that contain ingredients known to cause adverse effects may not be worth risking your health.

How to Avoid Skin Damage

Healthy-looking skin is one of your most valuable assets. Not only is clear and glowing skin attractive, but it makes you look and feel great. It can even build self-confidence and self-esteem. Your face is a statement to everyone you meet. Besides communicating how you think and feel, your skin can reveal such things as your diet and health. The good-looking have many perceived advantages. Persons of all ages who preserve a youthful appearance are likely to be more optimistic, outgoing, and social. They rate themselves higher in many psychological dimensions and are more successful in professional avenues. Finally, the psychological benefit of skin care cannot be over-estimated. Appearance is an important psychological factor for young and old alike because it counts heavily in human affairs.

Proper care can protect your skin from environmental damage and premature aging. This should include protection against UV radiation, and toxic chemicals in the environment, work place, and household. Second, proper nourishment of body and skin can help retain the youthful elasticity and even heal environmental damage caused by carelessness. No two individuals have exactly the same kind of skin. Each requires a personalized program of cleansing, toning, moisturizing, and protecting to maintain a healthy glow.

Your skin is the first line of defense against the outside world and as such is exposed daily to many environmental stresses that can cause irritation, premature aging, and even skin cancer. You can limit exposure to environmental and chemical damage to your skin by observing a few simple guidelines. The following sections give an outline of the most common sources of skin damage that can be avoided.

Avoid Harmful Cosmetic Chemicals

Fewer than four percent of manufacturers, packagers, and distributors file injury reports with the FDA due to cosmetic products. Only a few percent of injured consumers require hospital care or visit a physician's office after experiencing adverse reactions. The long-term effect of these chemicals on the rest of the population is unknown since neither the consumer nor the physician may associate a physical problem, particularly a systemic one, with the use of a cosmetic preparation. A much larger percentage of consumers stop using the product when they develop an adverse skin, hair, or eye reaction, and never report it to the manufacturer. There are several beneficial chemicals used in cosmetics that contain toxic byproducts stemming from the manufacturing process. Other classes of compounds may form toxic contaminants when mixed with cosmetic chemicals or when exposed to the air and sun (like those that form free radicals in the skin).

Consumers and cosmetic professionals alike are at a definite disadvantage when trying to avoid chemical stress to the skin and body unless they have the information on ingredients that cause adverse effects. This vital information is compiled in Appendix A, which contains a list of more than 460 cosmetic chemicals with known adverse effects. Also cited are the CTFA names of the chemicals, the adverse effect they produced, and references to the published medical publications. Check the lables of the cosmetic preparations you are now using. If one or more ingredients listed in Appendix A appear on the label you can minimize chemical stress to your skin by discontinuing the use of the product.

Avoid Environmental Stress

Solar radiation can be a damaging influence on your skin. The lower light spectrum which we perceive as light and heat waves have no damaging effect. Only the higher energy rays starting with near ultraviolet (UV) light cause damage. While the atmosphere prevents most of the higher energy rays from reaching us, enough of the ultraviolet rays penetrate the atmosphere to cause serious damage to our skin. The higher your elevation, the higher the intensity of exposure and damage to your skin. At an elevation of 5,000 feet (Denver) the intensity of ultraviolet rays is almost double compared to sea level.

The effect of UV radiation on the skin is called photoaging, as distinguished from intrinsic aging which is caused by the normal aging process. Histological studies (studies of functions and structures of human tissues) reveal several important changes in cells exposed to UV and higher energy radiation. First, sun exposure accelerates and exaggerates the clinical changes associated with advanced age. It causes coarse wrinkling, furrowing and elastosis (the degradation of the elastic material in the skin). Abnormal skin growths can appear due to changes in DNA by UV radiation, like solar keratosis, and the development of small, wart-like, red or flesh-colored growths on exposed parts of the body. These abnormal skin growths often develop into skin cancer and should be removed.

Another type of sun damage to your skin is caused by phototoxic and photoallergic substances that are put on the skin. These are otherwise harmless chemicals contained in cosmetic preparations or occupational chemicals that have penetrated your skin before solar exposure. When exposed to UV radiation these substances change their chemical structure and become allergens and toxins inside your body. There are many cosmetic chemicals in that category, including sunscreen agents and fragrance components. Some classic examples are musk ambrette and orange blossom oil. You can easily minimize damage to your skin from solar exposure by limiting the time you spend in direct sun-light and by using creams and lotions containing a sun screen that filter out the damaging part of the radiation. Unfortunately, some of these chemicals have damaging side effects that include photo-toxicity. These effects are discussed in the section on Sunscreens. The only way to avoid phototoxins is to identify them, and avoid products containing such substances. Tables A-1 and B-1 in the Appendix identify several of these chemicals.

Other environmental stresses are caused by pollutants in the air from industrial, automotive, and occupational chemicals. Our skin is constantly exposed to atmospheric ozone, carbon monoxide, nitrogen dioxide, sulfur dioxide and other chemical pollutants. A study done by Dr. Lester Packer of the University of California at Berkeley (November 1991) shows that atmospheric ozone considerably depleted the vitamin content of the skin. In addition, ozone can form peroxides (compounds containing reactive oxygen) that can destroy skin cells and cause premature aging of skin cells. Skin exposed to these atmospheric compounds can form carcinogenic nitrosamines. Frequent washing of the exposed skin areas and topically applied preparations containing vitamins can counteract this stress.

Anyone who works with chemicals in a warehouse or chemical laboratory should know the substances with which they may come in contact. The U.S. Department of Health and Human Services through the National Institute for Occupational Safety and Health (NIOSH) is required by law (Public Law 91-596) to publish a Registry of Toxic Effects of Chemical Substances (RTECS). The latest edition contains a description of almost 100,000 chemical compounds providing data on skin and eye irritation, mutation, reproductive effects, tumorigenic, and toxicity. It identifies thousands of chemical compounds that pose serious health hazards, although, to date, only a fraction of the listed compounds have been thoroughly tested. To find out about the toxicity of chemicals you work with on a daily basis consult the RTECS listing. Some public libraries carry a Compact Disc Read Only Memory (CD-ROM) version of the RTECS that can be searched with the aid of a computer.

The effects of exposure to environmental and occupational hazards to your skin can be minimized. Rinse the affected parts of your body often with plain water or mild detergent, if necessary. Most atmospheric pollutants are water soluble and can be easily removed that way. Also, use protective creams and wear protective clothing to prevent toxic substances from penetrating the skin while at the work place. The benefits of using vitamins in skin creams to combat atmospheric pollution can be found in the section on Vitamins.

Patch Testing

Patch testing is a convenient way to find out if your skin is sensitive to a certain product or ingredient. It does not, however, test systemic poisoning that may occur through the skin. It is also a quick way to find out if you are sensitive to certain emulsifiers, detergents, or essential oils before they can cause dermatitis. You can do a number of patch tests simultaneously. You only need to keep track of what chemical you put under which patch. Patch testing is a simple procedure using a simple round adhesive bandage with a non-stick pad. The pad is saturated with the substance to be tested and is placed on the inner forearm (or another convenient location) and left on for twelve to twenty-four hours. The patch is then taken off and the skin surface examined with a magnifying glass. If for any reason during the test the skin underneath the patch starts to itch or hurt the patch should be taken off immediately and the skin examined. No stronger reaction than reddening of the skin to small papules should be allowed to develop without seeing a doctor. For some individuals even the adhesive of the patch can cause a skin reaction.

Patch testing is mainly used for diagnosing the allergic or toxic sensitivity of an individual to certain chemical substances that can cause dermatitis (i.e., antigens, drugs, or cosmetics). Dermatologists use it frequently to determine the cause of dermatitis in patients so that the offending substance can be removed from the patients environment. Dermatitis and eczema are skin conditions that indicate a special inflammatory state. When dermatitis is caused by external substances, the resulting reaction is called contact dermatitis or contact eczema. There are two types of contact dermatitis, allergic and toxic. Allergic contact dermatitis is caused by allergens that trigger the immune system and is characterized by several stages of eruptions. First, the skin reddens, after which clusters of small pimples and swelling can appear. Weeping of the skin can occur as well as the formation of small blisters that lead to the formation of crusts. This eruption is usually accompanied by itching, which may vary from moderate to quiet severe. If the eruption becomes chronic, areas of the skin thicken and deepening of the normal skin lines and peeling may occur.

Toxic contact dermatitis may be provoked by repeated contact with toxic chemicals (cleansers, solvents, alkalis, and acids). Skin reactions to toxic substances can include some of the symptoms mentioned above (although the body's immune system is not involved). The skin may first redden, then drying and cracking occurs, and eczema and blisters may also develop. An example is dermatitis caused by surfactants (shampoos, foam baths, dishwashing liquids) and may have the following stages: reddening with increased swelling and formation of blisters, dryness to scaling of skin, and fine cracks in the skin to multiple fissures. Similar reactions occur with alkali (sodium hydroxide, ammonium hydroxide, thioglycolate, etc.).

The information in the preceding paragraphs is not intended to replace the services of a medical doctor but rather to give you a quick method of finding out if you are sensitive to a particular substance before its intended use. As an example, you may test your skin for sensitivity to rosemary oil which you intend to add to your bath water, or to find out if you are allergic to herbs you want to use in facial mask. If you have already developed a skin condition, the safest way to get relieve is to visit a dermatologist.

Skin Types

Since no two individuals are alike, there are as many types of skin as there are people. Skin type also changes with age. The water content of the skin declines from an average of 13 percent in a child to less than 7 percent for an older person. Oil secretion also decreases with age, especially in post- menopausal women because of the decrease in hormone production. Also, more than one type of skin may be present on your face. In cosmetic language this is called combination skin. This often occurs in the facial area called the T-Zone which consists of the central forehead, the nose, and the medial cheeks. The T-zone is often more dry or more oily than the rest of the face. There is no industry-standard classification of skin types. Each cosmetic company has its own system depending on the type of products offered and effectiveness claimed. There are, however, many similarities among them whereby skin types can be categorizided into a few groups. At the end of this chapter, you will find these groups listed in Table 11 under skin, normal etc., together with beneficial biological substances for your type of skin.

Normal Skin

Many young people (who do not have oily skin) and older people (who had oily skin in their youth) belong to this group. This type of skin causes few problems and is well-behaved. It requires careful daily care and environmental protection. The skin tone is clear and the pores are normal in size. It looks firm, supple, and free of deep tension lines and wrinkles. There are a large number of special cosmetic ingredients available for the preventive treatments to help maintain this ideal condition as long as possible. Among them are plant oils, phospholipids, herbal extracts and vitamins.

Dark Skin

Dark skin is biologically superior to light skin. It is more resistant to aging and skin cancer and is less prone to damage by UV light. However, two skin conditions of great concern to Afro-Americans are aggravated by cosmetic products. They are irregular pigmentation and scar formation. Several studies suggest that Afro-Americans in the United States spend a greater percentage of their income on skin grooming products than any other ethnic group, and that this may be due to their sensitivity to the presence of even minor skin blemishes. Products promising a cure from disorders of pigmentation (hyperpigmentation and depigmentation) and preparations for hair straightening are high on the shopping list. These and other cosmetic products have a high incidence of contact dermatitis and the formation of acne in dark-skinned people. As a result, hyperpigmentation is frequently experienced after acne or contact dermatitis have been controlled. Also, pomades used to straighten hair contain acne-promoting ingredients and can cause acne-like pimples and facial lesions on the forehead and temples.

Another concern is oiliness of the skin. There is no evidence that dark skin is oilier than light skin. Oil on dark skin is more obvious because light is so well reflected on a dark shiny surface. For this reason many facial cosmetic products that are formulated for Afro-Americans cause a reduction in oil normally dispersed over the skin. If used too frequently, these products may cause a deficiency of surface oils and damage the skin. Lecithin creams and lotions, however, reduce the oily appearance and at the same time nourish and protect the skin. Much research still needs to be done to better understand and treat the special skin problems of dark-skinned races. Dermatologists have had good results clearing up skin problems by simply discontinuing the use any cosmetic skin care preparations for a period of six months.

Dry Skin

The majority of middle-aged and older people have skin that is too dry. The primary cause of this condition is insufficient secretion of the sebaceous glands due to age. The natural hydrolipid mantle of the skin lacks the oil to bind enough water to keep the skin moist. This type of skin is tight and dry, and has often a flaky look with fine lines around the eyes, mouth, and nose. If this skin becomes dehydrated, it can look parched. Unless cared for properly, it usually shows wrinkles prematurely. Proper nourishment and daily care is indispensable for this type of skin. There are a large number of special cosmetic ingredients available to help alleviate dry skin conditions. Among them are special plant oils, like Jojoba oil, and those containing unsaturated oils, phospholipids, and vitamins. (See Table 11 reference "Skin, dry" for special ingredients for this type of skin.)

Oily Skin

Oily skin is mainly an attribute of youth since the abundantly present hormones are responsible for increased oil secretions of the sebaceous glands. This type of skin is shiny all over. Enlarged pores may be visible, particular in the T-zone. There may be scaliness with occasional blemishes around the nose, on the chin, between the eyebrows, and in the middle of the forehead. This type of skin usually just needs gentle cleansing and nourishing without adding additional lipids to the skin. Those with oily skin in youth will develop fewer wrinkles later in life. There are several natural substances, especially essential oils and herbal extracts, that reduce the excessive sebum production that causees oily skin.

Combination Skin

This expression refers to a skin that has one or more of the above skin types in different areas of the face. The customary combination skin type has a T-shaped area of oiliness across the forehead and down the center of the face. Caring for this skin type can be an annoyance because what works on one area may not work on another. Phospholipids, a component of lecithin, are valuable for this condition since they work equally well for different skin types. Many herbs and essential oils have the ability to regulate perspiration and sebum production. They promote or diminish these functions as necessary and can be found in the monographs describing herbs and essential oils in the special ingredients section.

Sensitive and Fragile Skin

This skin type is vulnerable and needs constant care. Signs of sensitive skin may be rashes, dryness, and broken surface capillaries. Sensitive skin must be treated with extra caution. It is usually fine and thin. It may turn red at the touch. It is particularly sensitive to changes in weather and is easily irritated by improper cosmetic ingredients. The skin can often feel itchy and tight. It also may have broken capillaries on the cheek near the nose. Sensitive skin can also feel soft and smooth one day, but dry and uncomfortable the next. If you have this type of skin you must be particularly careful in selecting the right cosmetic products and identify the particular ingredients that can irritate your skin. Fortunately, nature provides us with plant substances that are beneficial for sensitive skin and fragile or broken capillaries. (See Table 11 reference for "Skin, sensitive" and other related headings.)

Problem Skin

Problem skin can result from sensitivity to external substances like antigens and toxins, nutritional deficiencies, and systemic ailments. The resulting dermatitis is of three general types: seborrheic dermatitis, contact dermatitis, and photo dermatitis. Seborrheic dermatitis manifests itself as a red, scaly, itchy rash that develops on the face, scalp, chest, and back. On the scalp a light form of seborrheic dermatitis is most commonly known as dandruff and is further described in the chapter on hair care. It can be caused by stress, but its exact cause must be determined individually. Contact dermatitis has the same symptoms but is caused by substances that come in contact with the skin. It may also be a reaction in response to an antigen or by direct contact with a toxic substance. Many types of contact dermatitis, including acne, are caused by cosmetic chemicals. Photo dermatitis is caused by ultraviolet light and has been described in the section on sunscreens. There is a wealth of information available regarding the treatment of problem skin. Many of the recommended remedies have been used for ages. A number of physicians and dermatologists, like Dr. Jean Valnet of France, have spent a lifetime promoting natural healing methods. Table 11 lists over 50 specific indications that may help with your specific skin condition.

Acne

Acne is a form of seborrheic dermatitis and is the most common skin problem of young people. It is a chronic skin disorder that seems to be linked to increased hormone production during puberty. Acne can also be chemically induced and appear in all age groups. This condition is caused by over production of oil in the sebaceous gland and subsequent clogging of the pores and inflammation. In addition, the problem is usually aggravated by increased keratin production by the horny layer. Severe cases of acne can cause permanent scarring and should be treated by a dermatologist. Much can be done by proper cleansing and diet. Cosmetic ingredients that promote the formation of blackheads and acne and must be avoided (refer to Appendix A). Vitamin A and Vitamin B complex have been shown to control this condition. See Table 11 under "AntiAcne" for a list of special herbs, vitamins, and essential oils that have shown great promise in preventing and treating this condition.

Facial Care

The general principles of facial skin care are to follow common sense. The first step is to clean the skin thoroughly and to remove loose skin cells that are continually shed on the surface of the skin. The second step is to condition the skin with a toner and to restore the acid mantle that was removed by the cleansing process. The third treatment has a three-fold purpose. It must contain ingredients to nourish the skin and medicate if necessary, restore or strengthen the barrier function of the epidermis, and to protect the skin from environmental influences. The fourth and last step is to moisturize the skin and make it supple. Steps three and four are usually applied together. These steps should be completed before a make-up foundation is applied.

Facial Cleansers and Makeup Removers

The most important part of your skin-care program is cleansing and getting your face clean without stripping it of all its natural oils. Sometimes a mild soap is sufficient, especially if you have oily skin and use no make-up. Properly formulated cleansing creams and lotions are probably the most gentle way to cleanse the skin and are more effective than using soap and water. Facial cleansers consist of water, emollients, emulsifiers, surfactants and special ingredients. In addition, some abrasive substances, such as pumice or ground almond shells, may be incorporated as extra cleaning aids. These ingredients remove excess fat, sweat and dirt, makeup residues, and some naturally loosened keratinized cells from the epidermis. There are a number of chemical substances on the cosmetic market, called peeling substances, that aid in removing the top layer of keratinized cells from the horny layers. The newest addition to this group are natural substances, called alpha hydroxy acids. These are certain fruit acids that are said to gently remove loosened cells without mechanical scrubbing and which are especially suited for facial care.

During the cleansing process, the natural emulsion formed by the skin is removed. This leaves the skin vulnerable to any irritating ingredient that may be in subsequent treatments. The skin around the eyes is most sensitive and can easily be damaged by improper ingredients. After the facial cleansing process the protective mantle of the skin should be restored by subsequent treatments with a toner, moisturizer, and lubricant. Because the protective layer is missing after cleansing, the detergents used in facial cleansers and makeup removers must be non-irritating and extremely mild. They should be amphoteric with an almost neutral pH. The same applies to emulsifiers, and emollients, and any added special ingredients, like perfume. When applying abrasive material or scrub to the facial skin, remember that your horny layer has only a thickness of 20 keratinized cells or about one thousandth of an inch. Too frequent mechanical scrubbing can damage this important layer and make it more penetrable to unwanted substances.

The ratios of water, emollients, emulsifiers, and surfactants in a basic formulation for a facial cleanser are usually adjusted to fit different types of skin. A very oily skin may need a stronger surfactant or emulsifier for cleansing than dry skin. In recent years the difference between a cleanser and toner has diminished considerably. Most cleansers today contain special ingredients and active principles like herbal extracts, antibacterial substances, essential oils, and an increasing number of synthetic ingredients. Several dangers must be pointed out in using today's facial cleansing products. The first and foremost are detergents that have traditionally caused reddening of the skin and contact dermatitis, especially around the eyes. Emulsifiers and higher alcohols, like cetyl alcohol and propylene glycol and similar substances are next on this list. Another popular ingredient in cleansing creams and lotions is mineral oil and other similar ingredients, which aid in the formation of acne and which should be avoided. You should check the ingredient labels of all facial cleansing products before purchase to avoid compounds that can produce adverse effects. For special natural ingredients consult Table 11 under your specific skin conditions.

Toners

Toning your skin is a convenient method to remove the last traces of excess oils and old makeup, and temporarily restore the skin to its natural pH level. The application of a toner provides the opportunity for treatment of individual skin conditions. After cleansing, the skin is in a better condition to absorb treatment by active ingredients such as herbs, essential oils, vitamins, and phospholipids which have the ability to repair the epidermis when weakened by harsh detergents or other environmental influences. If your skin suffers from allergies or has dermatitis of any kind, antiinflammatory substances can be added to provide relief. If your skin and follicles are infected because of excessive sebum production, as in acne, ingredients that are antiseptic and control sebum production are particularly helpful. In addition, different skin types require different compositions of toners. With so many combinations possible, many formulations can be created including one that is right for you. The boundary between toners and nourishing creams and lotions is no longer sharply defined. There are many nourishing products that tone the skin and vice versa. To learn about the natural ingredients that are best for any particular skin, consult Table 11 which lists the different treatments for skin conditions you may experience.

Active ingredients in toners are used in small amounts and require a carrier fluid to be applied to the skin. Carrier fluids (except water) have their own effect on the skin. Alcohol in high concentrations is a skin irritant and should be avoided. Small concentrations of no more than about 10 percent are tolerated well and have the additional advantage of preserving the toner without the aid of commonly used irritating preservatives. Propylene glycol (PG) is frequently used as solvent for herbal extracts and should be avoided because it causes dermatitis in a relative high percentage of users. Emulsifiers and emollients are sometimes part of toning lotions and the same caveats apply as stated in the discussion of cleansing products. You should check the ingredient labels of all toning products before purchase and avoid ingredients that can produce adverse effects.

Masks and Related Treatments

The purpose of masks is similar to those of toners except that they give intensive care to the face within a relatively short period of time. Sometimes they also have cleansing and moisturizing properties. There is a different mask for every skin type and skin condition. They can contain a powder base of inert inorganic clays like kaolin, magnesium aluminum silicate, or bentonite. Peeling masks contain a synthetic resin that solidifies after application and can be later peeled off. Besides powder base and binders, masks can be formulated with a wealth of special substances, many of which have been listed in the special ingredients section.

Masks with a clay base are muddy pastes or viscous liquids that easily adhere to the facial skin after application. Clay has been a healing remedy in Europe for centuries. It is referred to as healing earth or healing clay. Clay has a large heat capacity and low thermal conductivity. Because of small particle size, a volume of clay represents an enormous surface area and can bind a large amount of liquid. These attributes are very important for applications of clay face masks. A thin layer of cool clay distributed on your face will extract heat from the skin and reduce inflammation. As the clay dries from the outside in, it draws all liquid and semi-liquid substances like water, sweat, oils, and toxins from the skin surface and beneath, and absorbs them. This deep-cleanses the skin and simultaneously acts as an astringent. With herbal ingredients, a properly formulated mask containing clay can make your skin feel fresh and renewed. Herbal powders are especially well suited as additions to clay masks. A list of herbs for nearly every skin condition can be found in Table 11.

Another method to apply intensive skin care is the facial steam bath. It is easy to apply and requires only a small washbasin or pan (holding about two quarts of water) and a large towel. First heat about two quarts of water to near boiling and pour it into the basin. Next, add the selected herbs and essential oils to the hot water. Place your face over the basin and put the towel over your head to enclose your head and washbasin. Keep your face at a comfortable distance from the hot water. The steam will open the pores and cleanse the skin. The selected herbal ingredients and essential oils will evaporate with the steam and produce the beneficial effect that you desire. After such a treatment the skin is relaxed, feels great, and has an increased moisture content. You can select herbs and oils that have astringent, antibacterial, or have other attributes (see Tables 7 and 8). If you suffer from a special facial skin condition see Table 11 to select the appropriate herbs or essential oils.

Nourishing and Moisturizing Creams and Lotions

After cleansing and toning you are ready for the most important step, nourishing your facial skin. The skin is nourished by countless numbers of small blood vessels that carry the necessary food, vitamins, and other necessities of life. However, because of today's polluted environment, dietary deficiencies, and influences causing accelerated aging, the supply of nourishment is often insufficient to keep the skin healthy. Each layer of the skin has different needs to function properly. The function of the epidermis (horny layer) is to protect the skin from harmful external influences. For this purpose it must be intact, healthy, moist, and well lubricated. Simultaneously, it must support the respiratory function by allowing the skin to breathe. A skin cream must support all of these functions without blocking the free passage of moisture, oxygen, and carbon dioxide in and out of the skin.

Phospholipids contained in lecithin can repair a depleted horny layer of human skin and restore its natural barrier capabilities. Phospholipids should be part of every nourishing cream since no other natural compound has this property. They restore the silky look to both skin and hair and are also moisturizers and emulsifiers. Naturally secreted sebum, under normal circumstances, is sufficient to lubricate the skin. But in today's soap-and-detergent happy society, additional lubrication is necessary, especially around the eyes since this part of the facial skin has few oil glands. An oil-in-water emulsion with 80 percent or more water supplies sufficient emollients to accomplish this task. Remember to avoid certain emulsifiers which can have adverse effects on your skin.

The next skin layer needing special attention is the basal layer. It contains the basal cells that are responsible for the continuous formation of new skin cells and renewal of the epidermis every 28 days. Today's environment is abundant with harmful chemical substances that adhere to the skin and penetrate even an intact horny layer. Once inside the skin they first affect the basal cells and prevent them from generating sufficient numbers of healthy new skin cells by depleting the necessary vitamins and other nutrients. They may even change the genetic code of the germinating cells and cause formation of tumors and malignant growths. Nourishing lotions can topically supply vitamins and antioxidants that are necessary for the generation of new and healthy cells and neutralize harmful chemicals.

Researchers have found that skin exposed to environmental air pollution, like ozone, shows a much lower vitamin content than unexposed skin. A study done by Dr. Lester Packer of the University of California at Berkeley (November 1991) showed that the atmospheric ozone considerably depleted the necessary vitamin content of the skin. Vitamin C, for instance, will counteract the formation of nitrosamines from nitrogen compounds that are present in the environment and which can lead to skin cancer. Fatty acids in emollients and emulsifiers can form free radicals that, with ozone, create destructive peroxides. Vitamin E is a powerful antioxidant that destroys free radicals that would otherwise go on a rampage and destroy skin cells. Vitamin A prevents acne formation and certain herbs reduce excessive sebum production (which is a major cause of acne). Among the many beneficial herbal substances are allantoin (a principle in comfrey) which helps to heal sunburned skin and bisabolol (contained in chamomile) that has antiinflammatory properties. Also, the moisture content of the skin is directly proportional to the content of essential fatty acids in the skin (arachidic, arachidonic, and linoleic acids). Emollients and phospholipids contain unsaturated essential fatty acid components and should therefore be part of any serious skin care preparation.

All the above ingredients need to be considered when formulating an effective nourishing cream. Cosmetic products that are fortified with those special ingredients mentioned are often not readily available but can be ordered from companies that specialize in personalized cosmetics. They can be manufactured for specific skin treatments, time of application (day or night) or environmental condition. All skin care lotions and creams are in the category of nourishing skin products. The following is a short description of their differences:

Day Creams and Lotions

Day creams are formulated so that they can be used under make-up. During the daytime you may work in an air-conditioned office with very low humidity. Under these conditions your skin will dry out sooner, therefore a product with extra moisturizers may be appropriate. If your occupation requires you to be outdoors frequently, you should choose a day cream or lotion that contains a sunscreen. You don't need to be in direct sunlight to be exposed to UV radiation since the rays scatter everywhere outdoors. Since many sunscreen ingredients cause adverse effects, be sure to do a patch test before using the product.

Night Creams and Lotions

Sleep is a fundamental human need and is necessary for the brain and metabolism to function efficiently. During sleep, the rate of metabolism, including that of the skin, slows down considerably. Night time is a chance for the skin to recover from the daily stresses. Because it doesn't need to be worn under makeup, a night cream or lotion can be rich in moisturizers, oils, and special ingredients. Since it will remain on the skin undisturbed for many hours, these nourishing and healing ingredients have a better chance to diffuse into the skin. When applying a night cream, use it sparingly to avoid disturbing the natural respiratory function of the skin. A thick layer of fatty cream causes water retention in the dermis and a swollen look in the morning. Also, be sure that no ingredients that are listed in Appendix A are present in your night cream. This is especially important because of the length of time that they are able to exert their harmful influence on your skin.

Specialty Creams and Lotions

There are a large number of specialty creams and lotions on the market. Few of them are different in basic composition from the ones already described in the facial skin care section. One of the important classes is medicated creams that treat acne, seborrheic, allergic and other skin conditions. Another class is sunscreen creams and lotions that are formulated as water-in-oil emulsion that do not easily wash off while swimming. Another example is protective or barrier creams for professional purposes. They form a film that protects the skin while working with harmful chemicals. Except for barrier creams and special added ingredients for specific treatments, all the above products should be similar in composition to creams described in the section on nourishing creams and lotions. Beneficial ingredients for the most common skin ailments and conditions are listed in Table 11. Products formulated with liposomes are able to carry these medicating or soothing substances inside the skin to make them more effective. Take special caution when using liposomes in specialty products since any toxic materials contained in the product may end up inside your skin cells.

All the above products are intended to be used together for your daily skin care regimen. Once you have cleansed and nourished the skin and restored the epidermal barrier, anything else that you may put on will cause less damage. After your nourishing and moisturizing treatment you are ready to apply a makeup product and to add colors. Exercise great care in choosing coloring products and check the ingredient labels to be able to avoid colors that have caused adverse effects in the past. Many Drug and Cosmetic (D&C) colors approved by the FDA are not harmless (see section on Colors ans Appendix B)

Body Care

A clean body is the basis for healthy skin. Bar soaps have been used to cleanse the body for hundreds of years. With the advent of modern synthetic chemistry, daily use of liquid and bar soaps is advertised as being good for us. What the advertisers don't tell you is that using these products strips the skin of its natural oils. Soaps and detergents should be used often, but only in small amounts and be of the non-irritating variety. Precious oils and perfumes have been used for thousands of years in tending the skin. Today, bodily care is not much different. The first step is to cleanse the skin thoroughly and remove loose skin cells that are continually shed by the horny layer. The second step is to nourish, moisturize, and lubricate the skin to make it supple. The regimen stated for facial skin care also holds true for the skin on the rest of your body.

Soaps

Water is a good cleanser by itself and is absolutely harmless while detergents and soap destroy the hydrolipid and acid mantle of the skin. It takes many hours for them to be restored, leaving the skin vulnerable to bacteria and harmful chemicals in the meantime. Bar soaps are chemical compounds made of sodium and different fatty acids (see the section on basic ingredients of soaps and shampoos). They sting a little when they get into your eyes because of the sodium ions that form when soap comes in contact with water. Liquid shower soaps and foam baths are formulated with synthetic surfactants that may not sting but, nevertheless, strip your skin of natural substances that are necessary to protect it from environmental influences.

There are a few surfactants that are skin-friendly (see the section on gentle cleansing). They are mostly amphoteric surfactants, and are partly made from natural substances like glucose, sucrose, and proteins. Their almost neutral pH makes it possible to add special ingredients to liquid soaps that would otherwise be destroyed by detergents and bar soaps that have an alkaline pH. The addition of certain essential oils can make these soaps antibacterial without the addition of synthetic biocides. Other essential oils and herbal extracts can soothe the skin and help relieve a variety of complaints. Foam baths are especially well suited for additions of herbal extracts. They can increase your emotional and physical well-being while gently revitalizing your whole body. Tables 11 and 12 summarize a wide variety of essential oils and herbal extracts with beneficial skin care properties that are compatible with such cleansing materials.

Body Creams and Lotions

Although the skin of the rest of the body is normally more protected from the environment than facial skin and the skin of the neck and arms, it nevertheless needs the same care and protection especially when exposed to a harsh environment for a prolonged time, such as working in the outdoors, playing on the beach, being in sea water or in a chlorinated pool or exposed to indoor and outdoor air pollution. Since nearly two percent of human respiration takes place through the skin, the pollution in an industrial environment or large population center (car exhausts) can affect the health of your skin and that of your whole body. Air pollution always increases the ozone level and the formation of toxic nitrogen compounds. Both of these compounds foster the formation of free radicals that cause irreversible changes in your skin. The regular use of creams, lotions, and bath oils containing radical scavengers, like Vitamin E compounds, help to combat this condition.

Body creams and lotions containing natural herbs and essential oils can provide many additional benefits. Minute quantities of antibacterial essential oils (lemon, orange, and tea-tree), when incorporated into body lotions, prevent odor formation. Some oils act to control excessive sweating or regulate sebum production. Some of these substances have been used for hundreds of years for the healing of skin ailments and others for the pure enjoyment of their fragrance. Since creams are part water and part oil, both oil soluble and water soluble natural ingredients can be added. Table 11 has a large selection of skin conditions and the natural ingredients which can bring enjoyment or relief.

Bath Oils for Skin Care

There is great interest by the cosmetic and medical community in the use of bath oils to provide skin care for the entire body. These are not the common bath oil preparations that coat your entire skin with mineral oil (which promotes acne), perfume, and little else. New formulations use the latest in skin care techniques to nourish, moisturize, lubricate, and treat the skin at the same time. The basic ingredients of these new formulations are natural emollients and phospholipids, that have a high content of essential fatty acids, and Vitamins. The superior moisturizing properties of phospholipids are well documented. In addition, they directly substitute for cellular phospholipids of the epidermis that have been removed through environmental causes (sun, pool water, sea water, detergents or surfactants) and restore its barrier function. This gives the entire skin a silky feel. The natural emollients not only lubricate dry skin but can also supply Vitamins to help eliminate free radicals, a major cause for premature skin aging and other symptoms. Together with phospholipids these bath oils contain unsaturated fatty acid compounds resulting in superior skin compatibility and deep moisturizing capability.

Since phospholipids are also natural emulsifiers, they finely disperse the oil and Vitamins in the bath water. They have a natural affinity for the skin, being a natural component of the cell membrane. After dissolving the excess oils and dross on your skin, they adhere firmly to the skin and perform their important nourishing and repair function. The same is true for any other oil-based ingredient like essential and herbal oils. They are the ideal skin treatment after a day on the beach, in the mountains, or after being exposed to environmental toxins. In addition to the effect of delightful fragrances and therapeutic essential oils, your skin feels fresh, clean, silky and protected without the cumbersome use of a lotion for your entire body. In addition, an entire range of natural ingredients are available that are antibacterial, antiinflammatory, antiperspirant, deodorant, rubefacient, and more. They can be formulated with a wide range of essential oils that not only have medicinal properties but contribute to your well-being as well. Consult Table 11 for essential oils that are applicable to specific skin conditions. Bath oils are especially well suited for aromatherapeutic treatments. A number of moods, states of mind and psyche are listed in Table 12 together with those fragrant essential oils that are reported to have therapeutic value.

Massage Oils

Massage oils should be formulated with natural oils. They may contain a special lecithin repair complex that will smooth the skin surface leaving it silky and soft. There is a large selection of medicinal and aromatherapeutic essential oils available as additives to help treat specific muscular or emotional conditions. Massage oils using rubefacient oils (i.e., rosemary) are being used to relieve muscular tension and pain. Specific oils with added vitamins have been used successfully in treating cellulite conditions. There are endless combinations of essential oils and oil soluble vitamins to treat your skin. Consult Tables 10 and 11 for possible additives.

Aromatherapy

Aromatherapy is very closely related to essential oils, fragrances, and the olfactory perception in human beings. The name aromatherapy was coined by R.M. Gattefosse, a French chemist and fragrance specialist, who wrote many books on the subject of cosmetic products and aromatherapy. Until recently his claims were dismissed by scientists. These findings are now receiving increased attention as more facts are discovered about how different odors affect human behavior. Pioneering research is now being conducted at several universities and medical schools in Europe. The healing properties of plant essences and essential oils were first successfully promoted in modern times by a French scientist, Dr. Jean Valnet, who published a classic book in this area called Aromatherapie (Reference 173).

The effect of plant essences on the human body is two-fold. There is a direct systemic effect, like that of any other drug, and an indirect effect throughout the olfactory system of the human body. Dr. Jean Valnet describes actual case histories of successfully treating cancer with plant essences. In addition, essential oils have been used for centuries in treating internal illnesses of the digestive tract, and in curing kidney and gall bladder stones. Essential oil molecules are very small and can easily pass through the epidermis to affect the entire body transdermally.

Essential oils can also greatly influence the mind and general well-being of a person. It has been established that the olfactory nerves are directly connected to the most primitive part of the brain. This brain system, called the limbic system, automatically regulates body functions (autonomic nervous system), emotional and sexual mechanisms, and sense of smell. All mammals (which include humans) release pheromones, a sexual olfactory substance, through special scent-producing glands. Many natural fragrances can mimic these pheromones and induce the release of a variety of hormones by the pituitary gland into the body. The connection between the olfactory and sexual systems take place automatically through the hypothalamic region. Consequently, perfume chemists include substances like civet, musk, castoreum and sandalwood (which are remarkably similar to the male human pheromone androsterol) in their products to make wearers irresistible.

The sense of smell acts almost on a subconscious level and is very sensitive. We can differentiate several hundred fragrances, but we have no proper vocabulary to adequately describe the odors. The part of the brain we are using for smell does not use the same logic as the intellectual brain because it appears to be a pure memory function. A certain smell can bring forth hidden memories and the deepest sensations of happiness, love, laughter, or terror.

Because of this direct connection of the olfactory system of the body to the primitive regions of the brain, aromatherapy has been called an open gate to our subconscious. The use of olfactory stimuli can not only be used for the cure of psychological disorders, but also to relieve ourselves from stress and anxieties by creating the atmosphere of joy and love in our own surroundings. Experimenting with different fragrances and combinations to explore our subconscious can be done with the aid of fragrant bath oils, foam baths, perfumes, perfumed creams, atomizers, perfumed candles, and incense. There is a wealth of literature available that lets you explore aromatherapy or psycho aromatherapy. Some of the most outstanding aromatherapeutic attributes of essential oils are compiled in Table 12 for your experimentation. For those of you who are interested in the art of psychic aromatherapy, a short description is included in Appendix B.

Table 11 Herbs, Essential Oils, and Vitamins for Skin and Hair Care

Condition	Plants	Essential Oils	Vitamins
Anti-acne	allantoin, birch, bisabolol. burdock, garlic, Jojoba	bergamot, camphor, cedarwood, chamomile, geranium, eucalyptus, juniper, lavender, melissa, palmarosa, patchouli, peppermint, rosemary, rosewood, sage, sandalwood, tea tree, thyme	Vitamin A (retinol), Vitamin B6 (pyridoxine)
Anti-aging	ginseng, gotu kola, hops, stinging nettle, phospholipids	frankincense, geranium, lavender, lemon, myrrh, neroli, patchouli, rose, sandalwood	Vitamin A (retinol), Vitamin B6 (pyridoxine), Carotene, Vitamin C, Vitamin E
Anti-allergy	chamomile	chamomile, melissa,	

Condition	Plants	Essential Oils	Vitamins
Anti-bacterial	aloe vera, burdock, chamomile, st. johnswort	bergamot, eucalyptus, geranium, juniper, lavender, lemon, melissa, orange, peppermint, rosewood, rosemary, tea tree, thyme, ylang ylang	
Anti-blotches	aloe vera, horse chestnut, st. johnswort	chamomile, geranium, lavender, lemon, ylang ylang	Vitamin C, Vitamin E
Anti-cellulite	allantoin, bisabolol, horse tail, plantain	cypress, geranium, juniper, rosemary, sage,	Vitamin C, Vitamin E
Anti-dandruff	burdock	carrotseed, cedarwood, frankincense, geranium, lavender, patchouli, rosemary, sage, tea tree	Biotin, Carotene, Vitamin B6 (pyridoxine),
Anti-fungal		bergamot, eucalyptus, geranium, juniper, lavender, lemon, melissa, orange, peppermint, rosewood, rosemary, tea tree, thyme, ylang ylang	

Condition	Plants	Essential Oils	Vitamins
Anti-inflammatory	aloe vera, althea, balm, bilberry, bisabolol, chamomile, horse chestnut, st. johnswort, witch hazel	benzoin, bergamot, cajeput, cedarwood, chamomile, eucalyptus, frankincense, fennel, geranium, hyssop, juniper, lavender, lemon, myrrh, neroli, niaouli, patchouli, peppermint, petitgrain, rose, sage, tea tree	Vitamin C, Vitamin E
Anti-wrinkle	ginseng, gotu kola, horse tail, phospholipids	carrotseed, cypress, fennel, frankincense, lemon, palmarosa, myrrh, neroli, palmarosa, patchouli, rose, sage, sandalwood	Vitamin A (retinol), Vitamin B6 (pyridoxine), Carotene, Vitamin C, Vitamin E
Antiperspirant	sage	benzoin, bergamot, cypress, eucalyptus, geranium, lavender, melissa, orange, peppermint, pine, rosemary, sage, spruce, thyme, ylang ylang	
Astringent	burdock, cucumber, sage, st. johnswort, witch hazel	bergamot, cedarwood, cypress, frankincense, geranium, juniper, lemon, myrrh, orange, rose, rosemary, sage, sandalwood	
Baby skin	balm, bilberry, horse chestnut, st. johnswort, witch hazel	chamomile, orange, rose,	

Condition	Plants	Essential Oils	Vitamins
Carcinogen blocker	aloe vera, burdock, calendula, garlic	cypress, garlic, geranium, lavender, sage	Vitamin C, Vitamin E, (tocopherol), Vitamin A, PABA (UV blocker)
Cell growth	ginseng, gotu kola	benzoin, palmarosa, rose,	Vitamin A (retinol), Vitamin B6 (pyridoxine), Carotene, Vitamin C, Vitamin E
Cellular tonic	ginseng, gotu kola, plantain, phospholipids	chamomile, benzoin, frankincense, cedarwood, geranium, lavender, myrrh, rosemary	Vitamin A (retinol), Vitamin B6 (pyridoxine), Carotene, Vitamin C, Vitamin E
Cellulitis	allantoin, aloe vera, althea, bisabolol, echinacea, horse chestnut, horse tail, marsh mallow, plantain	cypress, geranium, juniper, orange, rosemary, sage	Inositol, Vitamin E
Counter irritant	aloe vera, bisabolol, melissa	benzoin, chamomile, geranium, lavender, myrrh, patchouli, tea tree	
Damaged skin	allantoin, aloe vera, althea, echinacea, marsh mallow, plantain, witch hazel, phospholipids	benzoin, chamomile, geranium, lavender, lemon, patchouli, sage, sandalwood, ylang ylang	Vitamin A (retinol), Vitamin B6 (pyridoxine), Carotene, Vitamin C, Vitamin E
Dark circle	hops, stinging nettle	chamomile, lemon	Vitamin A (retinol), Vitamin B6 (pyridoxine), Carotene, Vitamin C, Vitamin E

Condition	Plants	Essential Oils	Vitamins
Deodorant	sage	benzoin, bergamot, cypress, eucalyptus, geranium, lavender, melissa, orange, peppermint, pine, rosemary, sage, spruce, thyme, ylang ylang	
Dermatitis, healing	allantoin, aloe vera, althea, echinacea, marsh mallow, melissa, plantain, witch hazel	benzoin, chamomile, cedarwood, geranium, jasmine, juniper, lavender, melissa, palmarosa, patchouli, peppermint, rosemary, sage, thyme	Vitamin A (retinol), Vitamin B6 (pyridoxine), Carotene, Vitamin C, Vitamin E
Eczema, healing	allantoin, aloe vera, althea, bisabolol, marsh mallow, plantain	chamomile, cedarwood, geranium, juniper, lavender, melissa, patchouli, rose, rosemary, sage, thyme, ylang ylang	Vitamin E
Eye lids, dry and inflamed	aloe, althea, balm, bisabolol, chamomile, horsetail	chamomile, geranium, lemon, thyme	Vitamin A (retinol), Vitamin B2 (riboflavine)
Fragile capillary	allantoin, aloe vera, horse chestnut, witch hazel	chamomile, juniper, neroli, rose	Vitamin C, Vitamin E, Vitamin E
Free radical scavenger			Vitamin C, Vitamin E, Vitamin E
Hair, blond	birch, burdock, calendula, chamomile, chestnut, clover, echinacea, horsetail, nettle,	lemon, sandalwood	Vitamin E, pantothenic acid

Condition	Plants	Essential Oils	Vitamins
Hair, brittle	birch, burdock, calendula, chamomile, chestnut, clover, echinacea, horsetail, nettle, phospholipids	benzoin, burdock, jojoba,	Vitamin E, pantothenic acid
Hair, dandruff	birch, burdock, calendula, chamomile, chestnut, clover, echinacea, horsetail, nettle,	cedarwood, cypress, eucalyptus, lemon, patchouli, sage, rosemary, tea-tree	Vitamin A (retinol), Vitamin B2 (riboflavine), Vitamin B3 (niacin), Vitamin B6 (pyridoxine), Biotin, Carotene, Vitamin C, Vitamin E, Pantothenic acid
Hair, dark	birch, burdock, calendula, chamomile, chestnut, clover, echinacea, horsetail, nettle,	rosemary, rosewood, sandalwood	Vitamin E, pantothenic acid
Hair, dry	birch, burdock, calendula, chamomile, chestnut, clover, echinacea, horsetail, nettle, phospholipids	benzoin, carrotseed, cedarwood, geranium, lavender, frankincense	Biotin, Vitamin E, Pantothenic acid
Hair, growth stimulant	aloe vera, birch, burdock, sage, stinging nettle, phospholipids	bay, cajeput, cedarwood, cypress, rosemary, sage, thyme, ylang ylang	Vitamin A (retinol), Vitamin B6 (pyridoxine), Carotene, Vitamin C, Vitamin E, Pantothenic acid

Condition	Plants	Essential Oils	Vitamins
Hair, light	birch, burdock, calendula, chamomile, chestnut, clover, echinacea, horsetail, nettle,	chamomile, lemon	Vitamin E, pantothenic acid
Hair, normal	birch, burdock, calendula, chamomile, chestnut, clover, echinacea, horsetail, nettle,	cedarwood, chamomile, carrotseed, cedarwood, cypress, lemon, lavender, rosemary, rosewood, sage, thyme	Vitamin E acetate, Vitamin E, pantothenic acid
Hair, oily	birch, burdock, calendula, chamomile, chestnut, clover, echinacea, horsetail, nettle,	bergamot, cedarwood, juniper, lavender, lemongrass, rosemary, cedarwood, sage, cypress	Biotin, Pantothenic acid
Healing	allantoin, aloe vera, althea, bisabolol, echinacea, horse chestnut, marsh mallow, plantain	benzoin, bergamot, chamomile, eucalyptus, fir, frankincense, lemon, myrrh, niaouli, thyme	Vitamin A (retinol), Vitamin B2 (riboflavine), Vitamin B3 (niacin), Vitamin B6 (pyridoxine), Biotin, Carotene, Vitamin C, Vitamin E acetate, Pantothenic acid
Herpes Zoster	plantain	bergamot, chamomile, geranium, lemon, melissa, rose, tea tree	Vitamin B12, Vitamin C
Insect repellant		cedarwood, cypress, eucalyptus, geranium, lavender, lemongrass, peppermint	
Massage, muscle pain		fennel, rosemary, thyme	Vitamin E

Condition	Plants	Essential Oils	Vitamins
Massage, rheumatic complaints		eucalyptus, fir, rosemary, sage, thyme	
nails, brittle		cypress, lemon	Biotin, Vitamin E, Pantothenic acid
nails, inflamed		cypress, tea tree	Biotin, Vitamin E, Pantothenic acid
Painful skin	aloe vera, althea, bilberry, bisabolol, chamomile, horse chestnut, melissa, st. johnswort, witch hazel	cajeput, neroli, petitgrain	Vitamin B2 (riboflavine), Vitamin B3 (niacin), Vitamin B6 (pyridoxine), Vitamin C, Vitamin E, Pantothenic acid
Perspiration		cypress, fir, sage, tea tree	Vitamin E
Pimples	allantoin, aloe vera, althea, bisabolol, echinacea, horse chestnut, marsh mallow, plantain	peppermint, tea tree	Vitamin A (retinol), Vitamin B2 (riboflavine), Vitamin B3 (niacin), Vitamin B6 (pyridoxine), Biotin, Carotene, Vitamin C, Vitamin E, Pantothenic acid
Pollution, environmental			Vitamin A (retinol), Vitamin B2 (riboflavine), Vitamin B3 (niacin), Vitamin B6 (pyridoxine), Biotin, Carotene, Vitamin C, Vitamin E, Pantothenic acid
Puffed eyed	chamomile	chamomile	Vitamin E

Condition	Plants	Essential Oils	Vitamins
Scalp treatment	birch, burdock, nettle, phospholipids	cedarwood, lavender, cypress, patchouli, rosemary, sage	Vitamin A (retinol), Vitamin B2 (riboflavine), Vitamin B3 (niacin), Vitamin B6 (pyridoxine), Biotin, Carotene, Vitamin C, Vitamin E, Pantothenic acid
Seborrhea	birch, bisabolol, burdock , calendula, horsetail, nettle	bergamot, cedarwood, cypress, juniper, lavender, lemon, myrrh, patchouli, sage	Vitamin A (retinol), Vitamin B2 (riboflavine), Vitamin B3 (niacin), Vitamin B6 (pyridoxine), Biotin, Carotene, Vitamin C, Vitamin E, Pantothenic acid
Sebum, normalizing	calendula, nettle, horsetail	bergamot, juniper, ylang ylang	Vitamin A (retinol), Vitamin B2 (riboflavine), Vitamin B3 (niacin), Vitamin B6 (pyridoxine), Biotin, Carotene, Vitamin C, Vitamin E, Pantothenic acid
Skin, aging	chamomile, ginseng, gotu kola, horse tail ; phospholipids	cypress, frankincense, lavender, myrrh, patchouli, rose	Vitamin A (retinol), Vitamin B2 (riboflavine), Vitamin B3 (niacin), Vitamin B6 (pyridoxine), Biotin, Carotene, Vitamin C, Vitamin E, Pantothenic acid
Skin, cracked, chapped	allantoin, aloe vera, althea, chamomile, echinacea, witch hazel; phospholipids	benzoin, chamomile, patchouli, sandalwood	Vitamin A, Vitamin B2 (riboflavine), Biotin, Vitamin E

Condition	Plants	Essential Oils	Vitamins
Skin, dry	aloe vera, mallow, plantain; phospholipids	jasmine, palmarosa, peppermint, rosemary, sandalwood, rose,	Vitamin A (retinol), Vitamin B3 (niacin), Vitamin E
Skin, itching	althea, chamomile, witch hazel	benzoin, cedarwood, chamomile, jasmine, lavender, lemon, peppermint,	Vitamin B3 (niacin), Vitamin B6 (pyridoxine)
Skin, normal	aloe vera, althea, bilberry, bisabolol, chamomile, horse chestnut, melissa, st. johnswort, witch hazel, phospholipids	bergamot, cedarwood, chamomile, geranium, jasmine, lavender, lemon, melissa, myrrh, neroli, orange, rose, rosewood, sandalwood, sage, ylang ylang	Vitamin A (retinol), Vitamin B2 (riboflavine), Vitamin B3 (niacin), Vitamin B6 (pyridoxine), Biotin, Carotene, Vitamin C, Vitamin E, Pantothenic acid
Skin, oily	birch, burdock, nettle; phospholipids	basil, bergamot, camphor, cypress, cedarwood, frankincense, geranium, lavender, lemon, peppermint, sage, thyme, ylang ylang	Vitamin B2 (riboflavine), Vitamin B3 (niacin), Vitamin B6 (pyridoxine), Biotin, Carotene, Vitamin C, Pantothenic acid
Skin, rashes	allantoin, aloe vera, althea, balm, chamomile, witch hazel	benzoin, chamomile, cedarwood, geranium, jasmine, juniper, lavender, melissa, palmarosa, patchouli, peppermint, rosemary, sage, thyme	Vitamin B3 (niacin), Vitamin B6 (pyridoxine)

Condition	Plants	Essential Oils	Vitamins
Skin, regeneration	ginseng, gotu kola, hops, stinging nettle	frankincense, frankincense, geranium, juniper, lavender, lemon, myrrh, neroli, patchouli, rose, sandalwood	Vitamin A (retinol), Vitamin B6 (pyridoxine), Carotene, Vitamin C, Vitamin E
Skin, relaxing	aloe vera, althea, bilberry, bisabolol, chamomile, horse chestnut, melissa, st. johnswort, witch hazel	bergamot, cedarwood, chamomile, jasmine, juniper, lavender, melissa, neroli, orange, patchouli, rose, rosewood, sandalwood, ylang ylang	
Skin, sensitive	balm, bilberry, horse chestnut, st. johnswort, witch hazel	bergamot, chamomile, jasmine, lemon, neroli, orange, rose, rosewood	Vitamin B6 (pyridoxine), Vitamin E
Skin, tightening	burdock, cucumber, sage, st. johnswort, witch hazel	chamomile, cypress, fennel, juniper, lemon, sage	Vitamin A (retinol), Vitamin B2 (riboflavine), Vitamin B3 (niacin), Vitamin B6 (pyridoxine), Biotin, Carotene, Vitamin C, Vitamin E, Pantothenic acid
Skin, toning	aloe vera, althea, bilberry, bisabolol, chamomile, horse chestnut, melissa, st. johnswort, witch hazel	clary sage, cypress, eucalyptus, fennel, geranium, jasmine, lemon, patchouli, peppermint,	Vitamin A (retinol), Vitamin B2 (riboflavine), Vitamin B3 (niacin), Vitamin B6 (pyridoxine), Biotin, Carotene, Vitamin C, Vitamin E, Pantothenic acid

Condition	Plants	Essential Oils	Vitamins
Sunburn, after	allantoin, aloe vera, althea, bisabolol, echinacea, horse chestnut, marsh mallow, plantain	benzoin, chamomile, cedarwood	Vitamin A palmitate, Vitamin C, Vitamin E (tocopherol), Vitamin E linoleate, Vitamin E
Sunburn, before	allantoin, aloe vera, althea, marsh mallow,		Vitamin A, Vitamin C, Vitamin E
Thinning hair, prevention	birch, burdock, sage, stinging nettle	bay, cajeput, cedarwood, cypress, rosemary, sage, thyme, ylang ylang	Vitamin A (retinol), Vitamin B6 (pyridoxine), Carotene, Vitamin C, Vitamin E, Pantothenic acid
Wrinkle treatment	chamomile, ginseng, gotu kola, horse tail	cypress, fennel, frankincense, lemon, palmarosa, myrrh, neroli, patchouli, rose, sage, sandalwood	Vitamin A (retinol), Vitamin B2 (riboflavine), Vitamin B3 (niacin), Vitamin B6 (pyridoxine), Biotin, Carotene, Vitamin C, Vitamin E, Pantothenic acid

Table 12 Essential Oils for Aromatherapy

State of mind	Essential oil fragrance
anger	german chamomile, roman chamomile, ylang ylang
anxiety	benzoin, bergamot, cedarwood, fir, jasmine, lemon, lime, patchouli, petitgrain, pine, rosewood, spruce
aphrodisiac	ginger, peppermint, pepper, sandalwood, savory, ylang ylang
beauty	jasmine, neroli, rose, ylang ylang

State of mind	Essential oil fragrance
calming	chamomile, lavender, marjoram,
celibacy	camphor, lavender
confidence	jasmine
confusion (relieve)	petitgrain
conscious mind (stimulate)	bay, black pepper, caraway, lavender, peppermint, rosemary,
courage	black pepper, clove, ginger, yarrow
depression (relieve)	clary sage, lemon balm (melissa), bergamot, sage, geranium, jasmine, lavender, lemon, lime, melissa, peppermint, petitgrain, rose, rosemary, sandalwood, spearmint, thyme, ylang ylang
emotional shock	melissa, neroli, rose
expectorant	cajeput, copaiba, eucalyptus, lavender, pine, hyssop
fatigue, nervous, intellectual	basil, clove, juniper, nutmeg
grief	melissa, neroli, rose
happiness	bergamot, lime, mandarin orange
healing	clove, eucalyptus, fir, myrrh, niaouli, palmarosa, pine, sandalwood, spearmint, spruce
health (maintain)	eucalyptus, fir, lavender, lemon, lemon balm, pine, spruce
hysteria	neroli, orange, tangerine
invigorating	rosemary, sage, pine
longevity	fennel, rosemary
love	cardamom, coriander, ginger, jasmine, lavender, palmarosa, rose, rosemary, yarrow, ylang ylang
memory	basil, clove, ginger, juniper, petitgrain, rose, rosemary
mental fatigue, strain	basil, caraway, ginger, peppermint, petitgrain, rosemary, sage, spearmint
mind	frankincense, myrrh

State of mind	Essential oil fragrance
nervous system	bergamot, cedarwood, cinnamon, cumin, fir, lemon, lime, pepper, peppermint, petitgrain, pine, sage, savory, spearmint, spruce, thyme
nervous tension	geranium, lavender, marjoram, melissa, neroli, orange, rose, tangerine, ylang ylang
nervousness	cistus, neroli, orange, tangerine, lemon
neurasthenia	lavender, melissa, patchouli, peppermint, rosemary, sage, spearmint, thyme
neurovegetative system	basil, ginger, lemon
peace	chamomile, ginger, jasmine, lavender, lemon balm, rose, ylang ylang
sadness	benzoin, jasmine, rose, rosewood
sex (aphrodisiac)	cardamom, ginger, jasmine, neroli, patchouli, rose, sandalwood, ylang ylang
sleep	bergamot, chamomile, celery, jasmine, lavender
spirituality	cedar, frankincense, gardenia, jasmine, myrrh, sandalwood
stress	cedarwood, fir, pine, spruce, ylang ylang

Chapter 5

Hair Care

In today's world, few things represent youth, self-image, and vanity more than hair and skin. When we feel good about our hair, we probably feel good about ourselves. We spend large sums on cosmetic products to shampoo, condition, perm, color, and style our hair. Many are horrified when they detect balding and will spend money on products, attempting to restore hair growth, that either don't work or have unwanted side effects. It is your heredity and general health that determine the basic condition of your hair. Internal ailments, the results of improper nutrition, and poisoning also leave their marks on your hair. Skilled physicians with the help of chemists can diagnose internal ailments, like mineral deficiencies and poisoning, through chemical hair analysis. Healthy hair growth is intimately connected to a healthy scalp and the overall health of the body.

Few people are satisfied with the way their natural hair looks. No other part of the body is manipulated or changed as much as hair. Luckily, hair is one of the most resilient parts of the body and capable of withstanding a great deal of stress and abuse and it continually replenishes itself. There are less stringent requirements put on hair-care products by the FDA than on skin-care products. Little consideration is given to the fact that hair growth starts deep within the dermis of the scalp, and the fact that carcinogens and mutagens (even in FDA approved hair colors, and other chemicals) can penetrate the skin to a certain degree, damage the follicles, and cause local and systemic adverse effects.

Function and Composition of Hair

A single hair is a complicated and intricate structure built by the hair follicles in the skin. It grows about one tenth of an inch a week. If your hair is one foot in length, it is probably more than two years old. Its thickness is less than a thousands of an inch and a healthy scalp has about 100,000 hairs. With that much hair it is normal to lose about a hundred a day, and an equivalent number start to grow daily from dormant follicles. Your genes determine the quantity, color, thickness, and texture (straight, wavy, or curly) of your hair. Our distant ancestors over a million years ago had a lot more bodily hair which, among other functions, protected them from the elements. Today, hair is mainly an adorning part of our body on which U.S. consumers spend over $3 billion dollars annually. The following is a short description of hair anatomy and how it is affected by cosmetic ingredients, both beneficial and harmful

Structure of Hair

The root of the hair is embedded in a tiny pit in the skin called a hair follicle that extends into the subcutaneous layer (see Fig. 83). The cells at the base of each follicle surround and fit over the papilla, forming a bulb-shaped root of the hair. The epidermal cells of the root proliferate, differentiate, and become keratinized. As more cells form, they are pushed up the follicle and the hair (a slender strand of keratinized epidermal cells) eventually pushes its way out onto the surface of the skin.

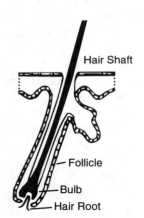

Fig. 83 *Hair follicle*

The color of the hair is determined by heredity. Special cells in the papilla, called melanocytes, control the color with the aid of a hormone secreted by the pituitary gland in the brain. As part of the advanced aging process, the number of pigment-producing cells in the hair follicles decreases, causing the hair to appear grey or white. At the start of the growth phase, the hair root stimulates the growth of a bulb and of a subsequent hair shaft. After that the hair grows about four-tenths of an inch per month. Each follicle has a sebaceous gland at the top that lubricates the hair. This gland has the important function of providing sebum for lubrication and flexibility to the hair shaft (the scalp produces about one gram of sebum per day). Each hair goes through an alternating period of growth and rest. For hair on the scalp, the growth phase can last over five years followed by a three-month rest phase after which a new hair begins to grow in the same follicle. Straight hair grows from almost round follicles whose cross section is also round. Curly hair is oval in cross section and grows from a highly curved follicle. The shape of the curl depends on the curve of the follicle. Finally, wavy hair is kidney shaped in cross section.

The hair shaft consists mainly of a protein called keratin. It forms from the up-growth of cells and keratin from the root. The hair shaft itself has three parts: skin (or cuticle), body (or cortex) and mark (or medulla). The cortex forms about 80 percent of the hair. It has a peculiar structure with at least four substructures. The cortex is made of fibrils that consist of many fine strands, called micro fibrils. The micro fibrils consist of the even smaller proto fibrils that are formed by the basic building block of hair, the alpha-helix (see Figure 84). A form of protein glue holds the whole structure together. Because of this structure, healthy, dry hair is extremely strong and can be stretched 30 to 40 percent without breaking. However, fully stretched hair loses its elasticity and will not return to its original shape.

To color or perm hair, the outer layers of the hair and the glue holding the fibrils together must be weakened to allow penetration of color and chemicals. Once weakened, the hair can never be restored to its original strength. The outer skin of the hair, called the cuticle, has five to ten layers of overlapping scales that make up about ten percent of the hair. They are arranged like fish scales (pointing toward the hair tips) and are held together by a glue-like substance. This layer is colorless and protects the cortex. On healthy, well-cared-for hair, these scales form a tight flat layer that reflects light and gives the hair a silky appearance. This layer can easily become damaged by mechanical (curling, pulling) or chemical means. The cuticle scales are chemically damaged when they are loosened with alkaline substances (like ammonium hydroxide) to allow chemicals to penetrate the cortex to bleach, dye, or perm the hair. This causes loose and partially detached scales that scatter light giving the hair a dull appearance (see Fig. 85).

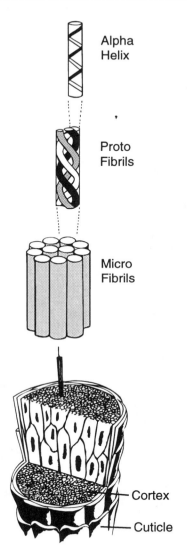

Alpha Helix

Proto Fibrils

Micro Fibrils

Cortex

Cuticle

Fig. 84 *Cross section of Hair*

How to Avoid Hair Damage

Proper care will keep hair healthy and beautiful. With the aid of cosmetics, hair can hide age better than any other part of the body. While you wear your skin throughout your life, hair is growing continuously and, depending on its length, will be part of your body for a short duration. The ends of medium-length hair may have been washed and brushed more than 1,000 times, permed ten times or more, and even colored a few times. No wonder that the ends of your hair are split, and your hair is frizzled, dull, and limp. Its structure has probably been damaged over a thousand times by harsh detergents, cosmetic chemicals, sun, and other environmental influences. Using the right kinds of detergents in hair shampoos, with additives that will strengthen the outer layers of hair, can minimize this damage.

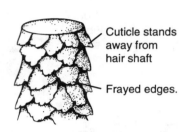

Cuticle stands away from hair shaft

Frayed edges.

Fig. 85 *Damaged cuticle layer of hair*

There are several types of scalp and hair. Each requires a personalized program of cleansing and conditioning. As with personalized skin care, no one product can satisfy the needs of all customers. Conventional companies mix shampoos and conditioners with few variations. They fail to inform their consumers in understandable terms what ingredients are present in their products and for what purpose. The only avenue for concerned consumers is to consult a reference guide, a cosmetic professional, or dermatologist for the latest information on which cosmetic ingredients may cause adverse effects and which are beneficial for a particular scalp, hair type, or environmental condition.

Minimize Daily Stress

The scalp is constantly exposed to environmental pollutants, and needs as much care as your facial skin. You need to protect your scalp and hair from premature aging and environmental damage. These are the same influences mentioned under skin care: UV radiation, toxic chemicals, air pollution, and household pollutants. Proper nourishment of the scalp can preserve youthful elasticity, and heal and repair environmental damage. Liposome products can revitalize your scalp, and natural repair complexes (phospholipids) can restore some strength to hair that has been damaged by harsh cosmetic chemicals.

Although the hair is not a living organism it has an intricate structure that can be easily damaged. Your hair can be damaged by mechanical (brushing) and chemical means and in the process lose its structural strength, color, and sheen. Heat can easily damage your hair through blow drying, hot combing, or use of a curling iron. Excessive exposure to the sun's rays dries out hair and makes it brittle (especially if has been previously damaged by a perm or dye). Wearing a hat or cap on the beach or in the mountains, therefore, makes great sense. Back combing or teasing your hair may cause breakage and overstretch the entangled hair when brushed afterwards. Metal clips, rubber bands, and curlers can also damage hair.

All parts of the hair are hygroscopic. Hair can absorb 20 percent of its weight in water and still feel dry to the touch. Hair with a high moisture content can easily be damaged through mechanical means. Avoid wet combing and brushing because it will overstretch the hair. Once overstretched, it will not return to its original length when dry and will lose its elasticity as well. Long hair is at a greater risk. Frequent cutting eliminates damaged hair. For long hair, the natural sebum generated by the sebaceous gland in the follicle can no longer reach the hair tips to provide lubrication and flexibility. Careful brushing, washing, and regular conditioning can help to prolong the useful life of the aging parts of long hair.

Chemical stress to your hair caused by cosmetic preparations is far more serious than mechanical stress. The principal stress factors in increasing order are detergents, hair coloring, and permanent waving. Shampoos cleanse hair by removing dirt, excessive fat, and scaling by means of surfactants. Surfactants, or surface active chemicals, are substances that foam in an aqueous solution and dissolve oil and keep it in fine dispersion. Modern chemistry has developed literally hundreds of different surfactants with varying degrees of effectiveness, most of which are damaging to your hair and skin. Many of them strip the cuticle of the natural sebum, removing lubrication and diminishing flexibility of the hair and damaging its surface. This process makes your hair appear dull. To counteract this damage a hair conditioner must be applied that coats the hair with another chemical compound (i.e. polymer resins) to restore the lost sheen. Fortunately, several surfactants are available that are extremely mild and still cleanse your hair sufficiently. They are identified in the section on surfactants and you can look for them on product labels.

Permanent coloring and permanent waving are the most damaging procedures that can be done to hair. Men and women are willing to sacrifice a great deal for a particular look. You don't necessarily need to discontinue these procedures but you should minimize the risks and control the damage. To clarify the damage process that takes place, the following is a brief description of what happens to your hair in the permanent waving process.

Effect of Permanents

The idea of permanent hair waving has been popular at least since the time of Louis XIV of France. The modern chemical method, known as the cold wave process, has been available since 1940. It applies two separate components successively, known as a waving fluid (alkaline solution) and fixation or neutralization fluid (acidic peroxide solution). The strong alkaline solution is used to break the polypeptide-amino acid link between the fibril strands of the cortex which gives the hair its strength and elasticity and which is also known as the disulfide or S-S bond. After the alkaline treatment the hair becomes limp and can be put into any desired shape. The fixation fluid partially restores the strength of the treated hair and makes the new shape permanent. The hair straightening process for Afro-American hair is similar except it sometimes uses sodium hydroxide as an alkaline solution which also permanently damages the hair and is toxic.

The process begins by pretreating the hair with an alkaline shampoo to strip off any oil and make the hair surface more permeable to the waving fluid. The hair is then set in curls with the aid of waving rods of varying diameter and wetted with the waving fluid (e.g. thioglycolate). The alkaline reaction opens the cuticle layer and swells the hair to almost 150 percent of its original size. This phase breaks the strong S-S bond of the keratin filaments and lasts from ten to 20 minutes. The thioglycolate solution is then removed thoroughly with a towel while the hair is still in curls. The fixation fluid is then applied to the hair. The acid reaction stops the action of the residual alkali and the hydrogen peroxide partially restores the S-S bond. Since this happens in the curled state of the hair, the curl becomes permanent. The fixation takes about 15 minutes. This process is not completely reversible and as result your hair loses 30 percent of its strength for every permanent wave application. Also, the fish-like scales of the cuticle seldom realign themselves smoothly, creating a dull appearance of the hair. Application of a conditioner soon after perming coats the hair shaft to give the temporary illusion of a smoother surface and to restore the sheen.

According to the U.S. Manufacturing File and FDA pilot study, permanent wave and hair straightening products are considered high risk since more than ten persons per thousand experience immediate skin and scalp problems. Little research has been done into possible systemic effects. The main ingredients responsible for these reactions are thioglycolate and sodium hydroxide. Both damage the skin and readily form compounds with chemicals containing heavy metals which produce toxins. There are many medical reports on nickel release and poisoning by thioglycolate due to stainless steel curlers.

Permanent waving, straightening, and coloring damage the structure of your hair. To minimize this effect, it is prudent to limit the frequency of these treatments. Because of the chemicals involved, a good hair care professional can help minimize damage and exposure to these chemicals. How tightly your hair is wound around the curlers, how the hair ends are treated, how strong a waving solution is used, and how well neutralization is done all directly impact the structural damage to your hair.

Effects of Hair Coloring

There are several types of hair colors, each with a specific composition and action mechanism. Hair restorers are hair dressings that gradually (after several days) darken grey hair to a brownish black color. The active ingredient is lead acetate and colloidal sulfur or sodium thiosulfate, which form black lead sulfate on the hair surface. Although still in use in the U.S., many countries have outlawed the use of lead for toxicological reasons. Lead is a systemic toxin. It can penetrate the scalp and has adverse cumulative systemic effects.

Vegetable hair dyes are now seldom used in the industrial nations except for Henna, a powdered leaf of Lawsonia Alba. The active ingredient is 2-hydroxy-1,4-naphthoquinone, which colors the hair in about an hour. It can be applied in an aqueous (hot water) paste made up of the dried leaves. The color obtained is reddish. It also can be mixed with indigo and other natural plant colors to produce brown to black color. Henna has caused hypersensitivity in some individuals.

Coal tar dyes are used for temporary hair dyes (washable after one shampooing), semi-permanent dyes (which will withstand 4-5 shampooing), and oxidation or permanent hair dyes. Temporary dyes are mainly part of hair color setting lotions. Semi-permanent dyes are formulated in shampoo bases. Direct colors are of small molecular size that ease the penetration into the hair cortex. Some of these dye ingredients are also part of permanent colors. Oxidation hair colors are the most important type. They are easily applied and the colors will withstand more than ten shampoos because the color is formed within the hair cortex.

In permanent coloring, two separate components of the preparation are mixed just before use. One part is a mixture containing the color intermediate and the other is a hydrogen peroxide or equivalent solution. The mixture is applied to the hair immediately after mixing. It also contains an alkali to soften the cuticle layers so that the chemicals can penetrate the cortex. Two different reactions occur in the hair at the same time: hydrogen peroxide bleaches the original hair melanin (bleached hair permits better coloring) and also forms a complex color within the hair cortex with the color intermediate. After about 15 minutes, when sufficient color has formed, the product is washed off.

Hair coloring products are graded as high risk with more than ten persons per thousand experiencing severe problems, according to the FDA U.S. Manufacturing File and a pilot study. Here, as in all the other studies conducted so far, the long-term effects of dyes have been neglected. Although the chemical stress to your hair due to the alkali used in permanent coloring certainly needs to be considered, the risk of permanently damaging your health due to the toxicity of hair dyes may be much greater. Researchers have determined that dyes do penetrate the scalp to a certain degree and get into the blood stream. As an example, phenylenediamines are still widely used in the U.S. as permanent hair colors despite being banned in European countries because many of them have caused cancer in animals.

Coal tar-based hair dyes, which are the majority of hair dyes used by men and women today, are exempted from the adulteration provisions of the 1938 Food, Drug and Cosmetic Act, the law that outlines the regulatory responsibility of the FDA. If a health hazard is established, the FDA cannot outlaw the product but can require warning labels to be placed on these products to advise customers of hazards associated with their use. After several studies by the National Cancer Institute and others it became apparent that many, if not all, tar-color compounds used for dyeing hair posed a serious health threat to the consumer. The FDA asked the cosmetic industry to voluntarily place the appropriate warning labels on such products. The industry has not complied because Congress has not enacted a law mandating such action.

During the last Congressional hearing on this matter (1979) it was learned that 150 out of 169 permanent hair dyes tested were mutagenic (cause birth defects when allowed to enter the blood stream) and that many of these were carcinogenic as well. Testimony on July 19, 1979, by the National Cancer Institute before the House Subcommittee on Oversight and Investigations of Interstate and Foreign Commerce on the Need for Cosmetic Safety

Table 13 Carcinogenic Hair Dyes

Carcinogenic Hair Dyes	
4-amino-2-nitrophenole	2-methoxyaniline
o-anisidine	4-methoxyaniline
2-chloro-p-phenylenediamine sulfate	4-methoxy-m-phenylenediamine
4-chloro-1,2-phenylenediamine	nitrilotriacetic acid
4-chloro-o-phenylenediamine	o-nitro-p-aminophenol
2,4-diaminoanisole sulfate	1,2-phenylenediamine
1,2-dichloroethane	o-phenylenediamine
Direct Blue 6	2,4-toluenediamine
Direct Black 38	

Table 14 Mutagenic Hair Dyes

Mutagenic hair dyes	
2-amino-4-nitrophenol	2-nitrophenylenediamine
2-amino-5-nitrophenol	4-nitro-o-phenylenediamine
2,4-diaminoanisol	m-phenylenediamine
2,5-diaminoanisol	o-phenylenediamine

Legislation showed the hair dyes listed in Table 13 to be carcinogens. In a hearing in the House of Representatives in 1978, certain hair dyes were identified to be mutagenic by a study performed by the Biochemistry Department of the University of California at Berkeley (see Table 14). Permanent hair colors in your supermarket are still being sold using these very colors compounds without warnings about their mutagenic or carcinogenic properties. In contrast, when the Japanese found that 2,4-toluenediamine (2,4-TDA) was a potent carcinogen, the Japanese industry slowly withdrew it from its market. When the cancer causing and mutagenic properties of the phenylenediamine compounds became known they were subsequently withdrawn from the market in Europe. The U.S. cosmetic industry has failed to act in similar fashion and the same dangerous compounds are still on the ingredient lists of the majority of hair color products sold today.

Another group of dangerous hair colorants are the hair restorers that gradually remove gray hair color using lead compounds as active principles. It is beyond comprehension why lead acetate is still permitted to be used in hair dyes when it is listed in the Department of Health and Human Services publication, Registry of Toxic Effects of Chemical Substances (RTECS No. 2474, 2475), as toxic, tumorigenic, and mutagenic. In contrast, the Swiss government has long ago outlawed the use of this type of ingredient in their country. I cannot give you a list of safe permanent hair colorants at this time because most of them are toxic in one way or another and their safety has not been established. Not even your professional cosmetologist or beautician knows what is in the hair coloring preparation they are using because no labeling requirement for wholesale products used in beauty salons has been mandated. If you must color your hair, do it infrequently and minimize skin contact with hair coloring compounds as much as possible. Know that your health is at risk.

Hair Types

Because the composition of hair is determined by your genes, there are as many different types of hair as there are people. Most of the differences can be grouped into a few categories determined by the physical structure of the hair, type of scalp, and the amount of oil that is produced by the sebaceous gland. Fine hair has a hair shaft with narrow diameter that may be due to a smaller width of the cortex or the medulla, or both. In most cases the innermost layer of the hair shaft is missing altogether. Because of the small diameter of the hair, fine hair is more prone to be damaged from blow drying and from chemical preparations used for perming, coloring and shampooing. Thick hair, having a larger diameter, can be harder to manage and needs extra time and care. Its follicles can be damaged easily by applying too much force when combing or brushing. Both types of hair can be further differentiated by the activity of the sebaceous glands in the scalp as follows:

Normal Hair

Normal hair has the optimum amount of natural oils to lubricate the hair strands and has an undamaged cuticle layer. This type of hair is probably extinct in the civilized world because all shampoos to a greater or lesser degree strip natural oils and damage the cuticle layer. In addition, coloring and perming generally weaken the shaft and the cuticle layer turning normal hair into the dry problem variety. There are a large number of special hair care ingredients available for the preventive treatments of normal hair to help maintain this ideal condition as long as possible. Among them are plant oils, phospholipids, and vitamins. See Table 11 under "Hair, normal" for special ingredients that positively influence this type of hair.

Afro-American Hair

The hair of Afro-Americans is substantially different from that of any other ethnic group. Caucasians have wavy or straight hair. Most Orientals and American Indians have straight hair with individual strands that are coarse, stiff, deep brown or black. Afro-Americans, on the other hand, have hair that is curled, has an asymmetric diameter (called beading), and is helical in structure because of the special curved shape of the follicles (see Fig. 86). This combination of beading, helical shape and curl makes the hair subject to spontaneous knotting. In the attempt to undo the knots, the hair is easily damaged or pulled out of the follicles. The hair appears to have no natural sheen because beading causes the light to scatter unevenly and make the hair appear dull. In addition, black hair is fragile, delicate, and dry.

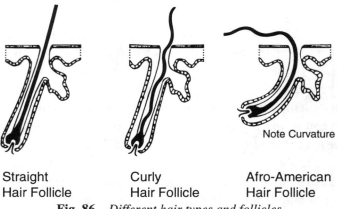

| Straight | Curly | Afro-American |
| Hair Follicle | Hair Follicle | Hair Follicle |

Fig. 86 *Different hair types and follicles*

Although the hair in its natural state looks beautiful, Afro-American men and women often wish to change its natural appearance and replace it with straight or wavy hair. During this process, Afro-American hair is damaged more than the hair of Caucasians, Orientals, or American Indians for many reasons. Hair straighteners (relaxers) consist mainly of sodium hydroxide, a strong alkali and toxic substance, that greatly weakens the already delicate black hair and scalp by causing irreversible damage to both. Hot comb straightening is another procedure that can cause severe damage and can produce second and third degree burns on the scalp. Scalp damage heals with the permanent loss of hair follicles. All these procedures, including oxidation coloring and bleaching, can leave Afro-American hair very brittle and prone to breaking. The simplest hair straighteners are pomades. They contain primarily paraffin and petrolatum with gums and perfumes added. Although they do not damage the hair, they often cause acne on the forehead and temples (pomade acne).

Afro-American hair must be treated very gently and, if it must be straightened or receive a soft wave curl, it should be treated by a competent beautician and afterwards treated with repair complexes. Afro-American hair is naturally very dry and with the addition of intense chemical treatments like chemical hair relaxing, soft curl permanent waving, thermal styling, and coloring, further drying results. You will find more information about special ingredients for dry hair in the next section and in Table 11.

Dry Hair

Naturally dry hair is due to low water content in the hair structure. Moisture in the hair is normally retained by a coating of sebum on each strand. If the sebaceous glands do not produce sufficient sebum, dry hair results. Naturally dry hair is rare among young people and can be helped by scalp massage, brushing, and scalp nourishment. Dry hair also can result from coloring, waving, or straightening. All these processes damage the cortex and hair cuticles which are a natural barrier preventing excessive moisture loss.

Another form of dryness manifests itself in older people. At the time the body starts losing the ability to produce pigment for the hair it also slows down sebum production in the oil glands of the scalp. In addition it can be observed that the follicles in older persons produce thicker strands of hair. All these conditions can make this type of hair become quite unmanageable. Dry hair is best treated first with a rich emollient shampoo to avoid stripping the hair of the little oil that is present. This should be followed by a conditioner that restores the barrier function of the cuticles and helps the cortex to retain moisture. Phospholipids can restore the natural barrier function of the cuticle and cortex. With a combination of phospholipids, natural oils, essential oils, and herbs, dry hair can be successfully treated without resorting to synthetic conditioning materials that damage the scalp and cause unwanted buildups. Table 11 lists a number of natural ingredients that are beneficial for dry hair and scalp.

Oily Hair

Oily hair results from increased activity of the sebaceous glands in the scalp. The oil production in these glands is controlled by hormones produced by the pituitary gland in the brain. Starting with puberty, the hormone production increases dramatically and can cause overproduction of sebum. As a result, both the skin and scalp become noticeably oilier. The hormone production and balance stabilize after puberty but the hair can remain prone to oiliness. As people with oily hair get older, the sebum production decreases naturally and the previous oily hair turns into normal hair that contains an optimum amount of natural oils.

Oily hair is usually very healthy and needs a shampoo specially formulated to remove excess oil and dirt without building up any conditioning ingredients. It should also be mild since oily hair is washed much more frequently than either normal or dry hair. Oily hair (of all the hair types) best withstands today's cosmetic stress due to shampooing and chemical treatments. Excessive oiliness of the scalp and hair can be positively influenced by a number natural ingredients. Check Table 11 under "Hair, oily" for a listing of these natural substances.

Dandruff

The living cells in the innermost part of the epidermis (basal layer) of the scalp rapidly divide and produce new cells. The transition from living to keratinized (dead) cells takes place in the middle part of the epidermis that consists of both living and dead cells. As the keratinized cells move to the outermost part of the epidermis they dry out and form the horny layer and are either worn off or fall off. This is normally an orderly process and regular brushing and shampooing will remove these dead cells from the scalp and dandruff flakes will not appear.

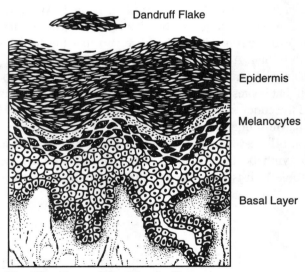

Fig. 87 *Formation of dandruff*

This orderly pattern of growth can be disturbed by a condition called hyper-keratinization, which means that too many cells of the epidermis are aging into their keratinized form and arrive at the scalp surface in dried form. They are too numerous and tightly packed to be removed by shampooing and brushing, and they stick together and fall off in flakes. This condition is called dandruff and is depicted in Figure 87. Different skin types produce different dandruff conditions.

When the skin is oily, the sebaceous glands produce too much oil that can irritate the basal skin cells around the hair follicle. This can cause an increase in new cell production and their rapid conversion into keratinized cells. These excess cells stick together and come loose in patches, and oily-scalp dandruff results. When the excess sebum production is brought under control, this type of dandruff will disappear. When the skin on the scalp is dry there is usually no overproduction of keratinized cells in the basal layer. The cause of this condition is not enough moisture to maintain the health and strength of the keratinized cells in the horny layer. They no longer can hold together and fall away as flakes. When the oil and water balance of the dry skin is corrected the dry-scalp dandruff will improve greatly.

Great care should be taken to select hair care products for dry skin that restore this water-oil balance. They should be void of surfactants and emulsifiers that irritate the skin and foster hyper keratinization, or dry out the skin. Some ingredients used in conditioners have this property and must be identified and avoided, as well as harsh chemicals and metal salts that are used in commercial dandruff products (see Appendix A). Some dandruff can be controlled by adding certain herbal extracts and essential oils to hair care products. Consult Table 11 under the heading "Hair, dandruff."

Basic Steps

Hair care is different from skin care in that it must provide care for the scalp as well as for the hair. Care for the scalp is essentially the same as that described in the skin care section, with the addition of special care for the follicles. Hair care is different since hair does not consist of living cells. Still, the same principles that apply to the horny layer of the skin also apply to hair since both of them consist of keratinized cells that need to be intact and well lubricated to perform their function properly.

The first step is to thoroughly clean the scalp and hair. This removes loose skin cells that are continuously shed on the surface of the scalp and removes dirt, fatty substances, and coating materials (from previous conditioning) from the hair. There are generally two methods to accomplish this: brushing and shampooing. The second step is to nourish and moisturize the scalp, restore and strengthen the epidermis, protect the scalp from environmental influences, and provide massage or medication (if necessary). The third and final step is to moisturize and repair the hair and restore the proper level of lubrication. Optionally, the hair can be coated with substances like proteins, gums or polymers, to give a special sheen and more body. This is especially necessary after intense chemical treatments, like chemical hair relaxing, soft curl permanent waving, thermal styling, and coloring.

Brushing

Only the first few inches of your hair benefit from the naturally secreted oil from the sebaceous glands in the hair follicles. The longer the hair, the less natural lubricant reaches the older part of the hair. Brushing your hair can accomplish the distribution of these oils and, simultaneously, remove dirt as well. The scalp also benefits in the process by getting a massage and by the removal of excess keratinized cells from its surface. Brushing must be done correctly to avoid needlessly straining the hair roots and to prevent hairs from being pulled out. A brush with natural bristles and rounded ends is best suited for this purpose. Bristles made from nylon or other synthetic plastics have sharp ends that can damage the hair and scalp surface. Long hair should be brushed in sections starting at the top, holding the hair firmly with your free hand to prevent undue strain on the follicles. Next, brush your hair and scalp from the nape of the neck to the top of your head. All this stimulates blood circulation in the scalp and guarantees that each hair root gets plenty of oxygen and nutrients to ensure a healthy life cycle. Don't forget to wash the brush frequently to remove rancid oils, dirt, and bacteria.

Scalp Massage and Conditioners

A healthy scalp is the foundation of healthy and well-behaved hair. The scalp is somewhat more protected than the facial skin but, nevertheless, needs similar care. Healthy hair is produced by healthy follicles, and healthy follicles are maintained by a steady flow of nutrients through the blood capillaries. If the circulation is poor and the blood cannot supply the follicles with sufficient nutrients and vitamins, waste products accumulate in the tissue, and the hair root suffers. Scalp massage should therefore be an important part of caring for your hair. Electric vibrators are especially convenient and are among the best ways to increase circulation. Although brushing provides some scalp massage when done correctly, a more thorough massage is needed at least twice a week.

Also, nourishing the scalp with vitamins and keeping the horny layer intact with natural phospholipids is an important task in order to prevent, as much as possible, penetration by harmful chemical compounds contained in cosmetic preparations and in the environment. Scalp conditioners are well suited to provide these important compounds and can be applied after brushing or after shampooing. They are usually formulated in a water-alcohol base but can contain oil-soluble as well as water-soluble vitamins. A wide variety of plant materials have beneficial properties that can control excess sebum production, inflammation, dandruff, and many other skin and hair conditions. Table 11 has a number of entries for different skin conditions together with herbs, essential oils, and vitamins to control them. Also, liposomes form well in lower concentrations of alcoholic solutions and can become carriers of these important substances into the dermal layers. Phospholipids can also repair and strengthen the cuticle layer of the hair and epidermis of the scalp. As with all products, check for irritating and toxic substances before applying.

Shampooing

Hair shampoos exclusively use synthetic surfactants as cleansing substances. Surfactants share the same fundamental molecular structure with conventional soaps and emulsifying agents. Among the large numbers of synthetic surfactants that are -manufactured today only a few are truly mild and non-irritating. Among them are derivatives of amino acid, glucose, and sucrose. Surfactants and soaps are described in greater detail in the section on soaps and shampoos as well as in the section on body care.

The most important function of shampoo is to clean the hair and scalp gently without stripping away all natural oils. Harsh detergents in shampoos not only deplete the scalp of oils and phospholipids (see Figures 28 and 29) but also harm the cuticle layer of the hair in similar fashion. Most detergents that foam are alkaline. They make the hair swell and the more alkaline they are, the more they will make the cuticles of the hair stand up. This makes the hair tangle and lose its sheen when dry. In addition, certain detergents (anionic surfactants) cause the cuticles to become negatively charged which cause fly-away and unmanageable hair. Your great-grandmother was probably not aware of the proper pH value but knew very well that after washing her hair with bar soap she needed to treat it with a vinegar rinse to make it manageable. Most detergents leave hair and skin at an alkaline pH that should be restored to an acidic pH with a conditioner.

Conditioning shampoos are a compromise formulation between the regular shampoos and a separate conditioner. They do not cleanse as well and cannot restore the acid balance because of their alkaline nature, but they can save time. They do contain ingredients that improve shine, impart softness, and add some body. Conditioning ingredients range from proteins, moisturizers, oils and waxes, herbal extracts, and vitamins. As with some skin care products, there is no sharp boundary between shampoos and conditioners. Special ingredients in conditioning shampoos and conditioners are the same with only a few exceptions, like pH adjusters or acidifiers, and body builders. Those shampoos formulated with amphoteric surfactants (of the type described in the section on gentle cleansing) do not chemically alter herbal principles, essential oils, and vitamins which can benefit a large number of scalp and hair conditions (see Table 11).

Conditioning

Unless you have oily hair, the hair is in bad shape after using a common shampoo, especially if your hair has been chemically treated. After shampooing, the pH of the hair is alkaline instead of acidic. The natural oils have been removed to a large extent and the cuticles of the hair are probably standing up as depicted in Figure 85. Left to dry in this condition the hair will tangle easily because of the raised cuticles, and will look dull for the same reason. Without sufficient oils on the hair shaft, there is no barrier to prevent moisture loss and the hair will dry out, become brittle, and break easily. These conditions are even worse if your hair has been colored or permed.

We have mentioned above that one quick fix is to rinse the hair with an acidic solution, like vinegar or lemon juice. This will help the cuticles to realign themselves with the shaft and make the hair shiny again. A smoother shaft also allows you to untangle the hair more easily. Next you need to repair the damaged cuticles, cuts, and split ends of the hair. This can be done by using phospholipids and proteins that will strengthen the moisture barrier and give the hair more sheen. Finally, some oil is needed to put back on the hair shaft to lubricate it and make it flexible. If you know how to make a natural mayonnaise, with vinegar or lemon juice, you can make a simple natural hair conditioner that has all the ingredients mentioned above. The egg supplies the protein and phospholipids for coating and moisturizing, the oil does the lubricating, and the vinegar or lemon juice will align the cuticles and reestablish the correct pH (not recommended with commercial mayonaise).

There are, of course, hundreds of synthetic and natural ingredients that cosmetic formulators use to accomplish these functions. These products are called creme rinses, instant conditioners, deep conditioners, hot oil treatments, body builders, hair repair treatments, and herbal rinses. They perform similar functions with varying effects on the hair and scalp. Most of the active ingredients provide more body to the hair by coating the hair with a translucent film that temporarily gives it sheen and seals in moisture. These coating materials are either oils, waxes, polymer resins, cellulose derivatives, or combinations thereof. Many of them cause a build-up on the hair that is difficult to remove and requires a strong detergent that in turn damages the hair. Conditioners also contain quaternary ammonium salts (quats), which attach themselves to freshly shampooed, damaged hair and neutralize the negative charge caused by harsh anionic surfactants. Quaternary ammonium compounds have been implicated in causing dermatitis and quaternium-15 has caused severe sensitivities to medical drugs.

Proteins are extensively used because they have a special affinity to hair. They cannot penetrate the cuticle and cortex and repair the hair, as is sometimes claimed, because of their large size, even when hydrolyzed. The only true hair repair complexes that penetrate the cuticle layer and cortex are phospholipids, certain vitamins, and essential oils. Herbal extracts, vitamins, and essential oils are increasingly used as alternatives to harmful hair conditioning ingredients. See Table 11 and the descriptions of herbs and essential oils for more detailed information.

Hair styling products are special conditioners that use liquid plastic (polymers) or similar ingredients to set the hair when wet or in curlers and keep it in the desired form after drying. They form a clear plastic film on each individual hair and protect it from moisture that would otherwise relax the hair. Most of these products are based on alcohol and water and have a tendency to build up a film that cannot be easily removed by mild shampoos. Because of the short exposure time of these products on skin and scalp they are rated low risk by the FDA. Always check the ingredient label since over 70 percent of hair conditioners on the market contain ingredients that have caused adverse effects in the past.

This concludes the brief treatment of Skin and Hair Care from the viewpoint of a scientist rather than that of a cosmetic practitioner. It is designed to help you avoid undue stress to your skin and hair by pointing out the hazards that are caused by our polluted environment and carelessly formulated cosmetic products. It also gives you an opportunity to follow the many suggestions of using natural substances in cosmetic preparations. I hope that by reading this book and avoiding harmful substances and procedures in skin and hair care, your look will improve and that you will live a healthier life.

Appendix A Cosmetic Chemicals Causing Adverse Effects

This is the first time that a list of this kind has been published. It identifies cosmetic ingredients that have caused adverse or toxic effects as documented by researchers and physicians around the world. By avoiding these ingredients you will have healthier skin and hair and avoid potential health risks due to long-term exposure to problem-causing compounds.

The name of a cosmetic chemical can be spelled in many different ways. The Cosmetic, Toiletry, and Fragrance Association (CTFA) has attempted to standardize the designation of chemical compounds. Over 90 percent of the cosmetics manufacturers adhere to the CTFA standard when labeling their products. However, these designations do not always correspond to the scientific names used by chemists and medical researchers when reporting their findings, but are usually very close. The entries in the following table are of either standard depending on the source of information.

There are several groups of compounds and many ingredients that contain or can form toxic contaminants.

— Ingredients that contain 1,4-dioxane (a carcinogen) include ethoxylated surface active agents (detergents, foaming agents, emulsifiers, and certain solvents). They are identifiable by the prefix or syllable "PEG," "polyethylene," "polyethylene glycol," "polyoxyethylene," "-eth-," or "-oxynol-."

— Cosmetic ingredients that contain or may form nitrosamines (carcinogens) include amines or amino derivatives, particularly diethanolamine (DEA) and triethanolamine (TEA). They can form nitrosamines when allowed to react with nitrosating agents that are frequently present in the environment, cosmetic products, or in your skin and body.

Ingredients listed with the designation "Group" following the ingredient name are of particular interest and importance. The medical or professional reference given identifies that this particular compound by itself or when chemically combined with other compounds can produce the stated adverse or toxic effects.

Table A-1 Cosmetic Chemicals Causing Adverse Effects

Cosmetic Chemical	Reference to Adverse Reaction
1,2-dibromo-2,4-dicyanobutane	causes contact eczema, Ref(47)
1,2-dichloroethane	found to be carcinogenic, Ref(153)
1,2-phenylenediamine	found to be carcinogenic, Ref(153)
1,4-dioxane (diethylene ether; 1,4-diethylene dioxide; diethylene oxide; dioxyethylene ether)	40% of commercial cosmetic product shown to contain up to 85 ppm of the carcinogen 1,4-dioxane, Ref(179)
	48% of cosmetic products containing polyethoxylated surfactants were found to contain 7.3 - 85.9 ppm of 1,4-dioxane. Ref(162)
	hazard: toxic by inhalation, absorbed by skin, a carcinogen; Ref(149 p.424)
	carcinogen contaminant of cosmetic products, Ref(93)
	carcinogen contaminant in cosmetic products, Ref(24)
2,4,5,7-tetraiodofluorescein disodium salt (FD&C red— No. 3)	cytotoxicity and genotoxicity established, Ref(63)
2,4-diaminoanisol	found to be mutagenic, Ref(154)
	carcinogen contaminants of cosmetic products, Ref(93)
2,4-diaminoanisole sulfate	found to be carcinogenic. Ref(153)
	shows decisive mutagenicity both on the X-chromosome and the RNA genes of the human male; mutagenic activity in metabolically active germ cells (spermatids and spermatocytes), Ref(107)
2,4-diaminotoluene (toluene-2,4-diamine)	carcinogen contaminant of cosmetic products, Ref(93)
	shows mutagenic properties, Ref(96)
	mutagenic activity in metabolically active germ cells (spermatids and spermatocytes), Ref(107)

Cosmetic Chemical	Reference to Adverse Reaction
	hazard: a carcinogen, Ref(149 p.1163)
2,4-toluenediamine	found to be carcinogenic, Ref(153)
2,5-diaminoanisol	found to be mutagenic, Ref(154)
2-bromo-2-nitropropane-1,3-diol	causes allergic contact dermatitis, Ref(88)
2-chloro-p-phenylenediamine sulfate	found to be carcinogenic, Ref(153)
2-ethoxyethyl-p-methoxy cinnamate (Cinoxate)	causes photosensitivity, Ref(152, 25.64)
2-hydroxy-4-methoxybenzo phenone	causes severe contact dermatitis in some individuals, Ref(176)
	causes severe contact dermatitis. Ref(164)
2-methoxy-5-methyl-4-nitrobenzenamine	found as contaminant in FD&C red no. 40, Ref(43)
2-methoxyaniline	found to be carcinogenic, Ref(153)
2-methyl-4-isothiazolin-3-one	causes contact dermatitis, Ref(21)
	causes contact allergies, Ref(33)
2-nitro-4-phenylenediamine	carcinogen contaminants of cosmetic products, Ref(93)
	carcinogen contaminants of cosmetic products, Ref(93)
	shows mutagenic properties, Ref(101)
	found to be carcinogenic, Ref(153)
	found to be mutagenic, Ref(154)
2-nitropropane	carcinogen, systemic effects, Ref(116)
	hazard: carcinogen, Ref(149 p.832)
2-phenoxyethanol (ethylene glycol monophenyl ether)	causes allergic reactions, Ref(186)
	causes chemically induced contact dermatitis, Ref(4)
2-tert-butylhydroquinone	causes allergic contact dermatitis, Ref(74)
	causes allergic contact dermatitis (in lip gloss), Ref(80)

Cosmetic Chemical	Reference to Adverse Reaction
	causes contact dermatitis (in lipstick), Ref(94)
3-carbethoxypsoralen	phototoxin; reacts with UV radiation to yield genotoxin, Ref(19)
3-methyl isothiazolin	causes contact allergies, Ref(33)
4,5,8-trimethylpsoralen	phototoxin; reacts with UV radiation to yield genotoxin, Ref(19)
4-chloro-1,2-phenylenediamine	found to be carcinogenic, Ref(153)
4-isopropyl-dibenzoylmethane	causes contact dermatitis, Ref(44)
4-methoxy-3-phenylenediamine	carcinogen contaminants of cosmetic products, Ref(93)
4-methoxy-m-phenylene diamine	found to be carcinogenic, Ref(153)
4-methoxyaniline	found to be carcinogenic, Ref(153)
4-nitro-o-phenylenediamine (4-NOPD)	found to be mutagenic, Ref(154)
	shows mutagenic properties, Ref(101)
	shows decisive mutagenicity both on the X-chromosome and the RNA genes of the human male, Ref(106)
5,7-dihydroxy-4-methyl coumarin	found to be a skin sensitizer, Ref(42)
5,7-dihydroxycoumarin	found to be a skin sensitizer, Ref(42)
5-chloro-2-methyl-4-iso thiazolin-3-one	causes contact dermatitis, Ref(21)
	causes contact allergies, Ref(33)
5-chloro-3-methyl isothiazolone	causes contact allergies, Ref(33)
5-methoxypsoralen	phototoxin; reacts with UV radiation to yield genotoxin, Ref(19)
	causes cutaneous phototoxicity reactions, Ref(66)
6-methylquinophthalone	causes dermatitis, Ref(105)
7-methylpyrido[3,4-c]psoralen	phototoxin; reacts with UV radiation to yield genotoxin, Ref(19)
8-methoxypsoralen (methoxsalen)	phototoxin; reacts with UV radiation to yield genotoxin, Ref(19)
	causes cutaneous phototoxicity reactions, Ref(66)

Cosmetic Chemical	Reference to Adverse Reaction
acetyl ethyl tetramethyl tetralin (AETT)	can produce hyperirretability and other system effects, Ref(98)
alcohols and polyols "Group"	causes contact dermatitis Ref(90)
alkanoamides "Group"	nitrosamines can form in all cosmetic ingredients containing amines and amino derivatives with nitrogen compounds, Ref(150); note: nitrosamines are known carcinogens, Ref(16) & causes allergic reactions and contact dermatitis, Ref(75)
alkoxylated alcohols "Group"	may contain dangerous levels of dioxane, a potent toxin, as a manufacturing byproduct, Ref(150)
alkoxylated amides "Group"	nitrosamines can form in all cosmetic ingredients containing amines and amino derivatives with nitrogen compounds, Ref(150); note: nitrosamines are known carcinogens, Ref(16) & causes allergic reactions and contact dermatitis, Ref(75)
alkoxylated amines "Group"	may contain dangerous levels of ethylen oxide and/or dioxane, both potent toxins, as a manufacturing byproduct, Ref(150)
alkoxylated carboxylic acids "Group"	may contain dangerous levels of ethylen oxide and/or dioxane, both potent toxins, as a manufacturing byproduct, Ref(150)
alkyl ether sulfates "Group"	nitrosamines can form in all cosmetic ingredients containing amines and amino derivatives with nitrogen compounds, Ref(150); note: nitrosamines are known carcinogens, Ref(16) & causes allergic reactions and contact dermatitis, Ref(75)
alkyl sulfates "Group"	causes skin irritation and dermatitis, Ref(100)
alpha-pinene	causes contact dermatitis, Ref(76)
	hazard: skin irritant, Ref(149 p.920)

Cosmetic Chemical	Reference to Adverse Reaction
amine "Group"	nitrosamines can form in all cosmetic ingredients containing amines and amino derivatives with nitrogen compounds, Ref(150); note: nitrosamines are known carcinogens, Ref(16) & causes allergic reactions and contact dermatitis, Ref(75)
ammonium chloride	causes severe eye and skin irritation, Ref(175)
anthanthrene	carcinogen contaminant in mineral oil, Ref(95)
benzalkonium chloride (quaternary ammonium compound)	hazard: highly toxic, Ref(149 p.128)
benzamidines "Group"	causes facial dermatoses and contact dermatitis, Ref(39)
benzo-a-pyrene	carcinogen contaminant in mineral oil, Ref(197)
benzo-b-fluroanthene	carcinogen contaminant in mineral oil, Ref(197)
benzoates "Group"	causes contact dermatitis, Ref(44)
	causes inflammatory reaction in rabbits; toxicity. Ref(53)
benzocaine (ethyl-p-aminobenzoate)	causes contact dermatitis. Ref(17)
	hazard: toxic by ingestion. Ref(149 p.478)
benzoic acid (carboxbenzene; benzenecarboxylic acid; phenylformic acid)	causes allergic reactions. Ref(89)
	toxic by ingestion, Ref(149 p.132)
benzoic acid n-alkyl esters	causes inflammatory reaction in rabbits, Ref(53)
benzoin (bitter almond-oil camphor; benzoylphenyl carbinol; 2-hydroxy-2-phenylacetophenone; phenylbenzoyl carbinol)	hazard: highly toxic, Ref(149 p.132)
	causes contact dermatitis, ref(104)

Cosmetic Chemical	Reference to Adverse Reaction
benzophenone-n	causes severe contact dermatitis in some individuals, Ref(188)
	causes photosensitivity, Ref(152, 25.64)
benzophenone-n (1-12) (diphenylketone)	causes contact dermatitis, Ref(117)
benzophenones "Group"	causes severe contact dermatitis, Ref(164)
benzyl alcohol (alpha-hydroxytoluene; phenylmethanol; phenylcarbinol)	causes contact dermatitis, Ref(118)
	hazard: highly toxic, Ref(149 p.134)
benzyl benzoate	causes allergic reactions, Ref(89)
	causes eye and skin irritation, Ref(149 p.135)
benzylparaben	shown to have low sensitizing potential at low concentrations, Ref(56)
bergamot oil	causes contact dermatitis, Ref(76)
BHA (butylated hydroxyanisole)	causes allergic contact dermatitis, Ref(74)
	hazard: toxic by ingestion. Use in foods restricted. Ref(149 p.183)
BHT (butylated hydroxytoluene)	found to be carcinogenic, Ref(153)
	causes allergic contact dermatitis, Ref(74)
bismuth	causes intellectual impairment and memory loss punctuated by periods of confusion, tremulousness, clumsiness, difficulty in walking, and myoclonic jerks, Ref(112)
blue No. 99	causes contact dermatitis, Ref(27)
boranes	highly toxic, Ref(149 p.161)
boranes "Group"	causes contact allergies; other adverse effects, Ref(48)
boric acids "Group"	causes fetal malformations and fetal death in mice, Ref(157)
bornelone	causes contact allergies, Ref(48)
bronopol	causes contact allergies, Ref(35)

Cosmetic Chemical	Reference to Adverse Reaction
	Induced contact dermatitis, Ref(65)
	causes dermatitis, Ref(89)
butanol	causes skin and eye inflammation, Ref(116)
butyl acetate	causes skin and respiratory irritations, Ref(116)
	hazard: skin irritant, toxic, Ref(149 p.181)
butyl alcohol	causes skin and eye inflammation, Ref(116)
butyl stearate (butyl octadecanoate)	shown to have comedogenic (acne promoting) properties, Ref(82)
	has acneigenic properties, Ref(130)
butylated hydroxyanisole "Group"	causes allergic contact dermatitis; adverse effects, Ref(74)
butylated hydroxyanisole (BHA)	causes allergic contact dermatitis, Ref(74)
butylated hydroxytoluene	found to be carcinogenic, Ref(153)
butylated hydroxytoluene "Group"	causes allergic contact dermatitis; adverse effects, Ref(74)
butylhydroxyanisol	causes allergic reactions, Ref(89)
butylparaben (n-butyl hydroxybenzoate)	shown to have low sensitizing potential at low concentrations, Ref(56)
	causes systemic eczematous, contact dermatitis and angry back, Ref(122,123,124,25)
cacao, butter of (theobroma oil, cocoa butter)	causes follicular hyperkeratosis (chemically induced acne), Ref(72)
calendula extract	causes irritant dermatitis from plant and tincture, Ref(120 p.317)
canthaxanthin	causes fatal (death) aplastic anemia, Ref(20)
	hazard: oral intake may cause loss of night vision, Ref(149 p.213)
carba-mix	causes contact dermatitis, Ref(17)

Cosmetic Chemical	Reference to Adverse Reaction
carotene derivatives, non-provitamin A	reduction of red blood cells production, Ref(20)
	irreversible damage to retina, Ref(216)
carotene, synthetic (provitamin A)	causes fatal (death) aplastic anemia, Ref(20)
carrot extract	is a photo sensitizer, Ref(120)
castor oil (ricinus oil)	causes allergic cheilitis in lipsticks, Ref(11)
cetearyl alcohol	causes contact sensitivity and dermatitis, Ref(134)
ceteth-n (1-45)	may contain dangerous levels of ethylen oxide and/or dioxane, both potent toxins, as a manufacturing byproduct, Ref(150)
cetyl alcohol (alcohol C-16; cetylic alcohol; 1-hexadecanol, normal; primary hexadecyl alcohol; palmityl alcohol)	causes contact eczema, Ref(100)
cetyl stearyl alcohol	causes contact dermatitis, Ref(26)
chamomile extract	causes allergic dermatitis in creams, Ref(120)
chloracetamide	causes cosmetic dermatitis, Ref(71)
chloracetamide	causes allergic reactions, Ref(89)
chloramphenicol	causes contact eczema, Ref(100)
	hazard: has deleterious and dangerous side effects, must conform to FDA labeling requirements, use is closely restricted, Ref(149 p.257)
chloromethylisothiazolinone	causes contact dermatitis, Ref(17)
chloropromazine "Group"	causes cutaneous phototoxicity reactions; adverse effects, Ref(66)
choleth-n	may contain dangerous levels of ethylen oxide and/or dioxane, both potent toxins, as a manufacturing byproduct, Ref(150)
chromates	contact allergen, Ref(46)
	causes contact dermatitis, Ref(17)

Cosmetic Chemical	Reference to Adverse Reaction
cinnamates "Group"	causes stinging sensations; adverse effects, Ref(103)
cinnamic aldehyde (cinnamaldehyde; 3-phenylpropenal;cinnamyl aldehyde)	causes contact dermatitis, Ref(23)
Cinoxate (2-ethoxyethyl-p-methoxy cinnamate)	causes photosensitivity, Ref(152, 25, 64)
clove oil (caryophyllus oil)	weak sensitizer, Ref(120)
coal tar derivatives "Group" (coal tar pitch volatiles)	shown to have comedogenic (acne promoting) properties, Ref(82)
	hazard: A human carcinogen, toxic by inhalation, Ref(149 p.290)
cobalt	causes contact dermatitis, Ref(17)
	hazard: toxic by inhalation, Ref(149 p.291)
cocamide DEA (cocamide diethanolamine)	nitrosamines can form in all cosmetic ingredients containing amines and amino derivatives with nitrogen compounds, Ref(150); note: nitrosamines are known carcinogens, Ref(16) & causes allergic reactions and contact dermatitis, Ref(75)
cocamide MEA (cocamide monoethanolamine)	nitrosamines can form in all cosmetic ingredients containing amines and amino derivatives with nitrogen compounds, Ref(150); note: nitrosamines are known carcinogens, Ref(16) & causes allergic reactions and contact dermatitis, Ref(75)
cocamide MIPA (cocamide monoisopropanolamine)	nitrosamines can form in all cosmetic ingredients containing amines and amino derivatives with nitrogen compounds, Ref(150); note: nitrosamines are known carcinogens, Ref(16); causes allergic reactions and contact dermatitis, Ref(75)
cocamidopropyl betaine	causes eyelid dermatitis, Ref(8)
cocoa butter (theobroma oil, cacao butter)	shown to promote acne, Ref(72)
coconut oil	contains skin irritants (caproic-,caprylic-,capric acids), Ref(120)

Cosmetic Chemical	Reference to Adverse Reaction
colophony (synonym for rosin)	causes eyelid dermatitis, Ref(172)
	causes allergic reactions, Ref(54)
comfrey extract	leaves have irritant properties, Ref(120)
corn oil (maize oil)	has acneigenic properties, Ref(130)
cornflower distillate	causes allergy and photosensitivity-, Ref(120)
cornflower extract	causes allergy and photosensitivity-, Ref(120)
coumarin (cumarin; benzopyrone; tonka bean camphor)	hazard: toxic by ingestion; carcinogenic, use in food products prohibited (FDA), Ref(149 p.318)
coumarin "Group"	found to be skin sensitizer; adverse effects, Ref(42)
cyanide "Group"	causes poisoning from a cosmetic nail remover, Ref(14)
cycloheximide	inhibits skin cell metabolism (lips), Ref(2)
	toxic by ingestion, Ref(149 p.336)
DEA (diethanolamine)	hazard: toxic, Ref(149 p.386)
	nitrosamines can form in all cosmetic ingredients containing amines and amino derivatives with nitrogen compounds, Ref(150); note: nitrosamines are known carcinogens, Ref(16)
DEA cetyl phosphate	nitrosamines can form in all cosmetic ingredients containing amines and amino derivatives with nitrogen compounds, Ref(150); note: nitrosamines are known carcinogens, Ref(16)
DEA dihydroxypalmityl phosphate	causes contact allergies, Ref(61)
DEA lauryl sulfate	nitrosamines can form in all cosmetic ingredients containing amines and amino derivatives with nitrogen compounds, Ref(150); note: nitrosamines are known carcinogens, Ref(16)
DEA methoxycinnamate	can form cancer causes nitrosoamines in sunlight (photo toxin), Ref(150)

Cosmetic Chemical	Reference to Adverse Reaction
decyl oleate	has comedogenic (acne promoting) properties, Ref(82)
diamine (hydrazine)	hazard: toxic by ingestion, inhalation, and skin absorption; strong irritant to skin and eyes; a carcinogen (OSHA), Ref(149 p.612)
diamines "Group" (hydrazine)	mutagenic and carcinogenic properties; adverse effects, Ref(91)
diammonium dithiodiglycolate	causes eczema and contact dermatitis, Ref(144)
diazolidinyl urea	causes contact dermatitis, Ref(34)
	causes dermatitis, Ref(46)
dibromocyanobutane (Tektamer 38)	causes allergic contact dermatitis, Ref(180)
	causes allergic contact dermatitis, Ref(5)
dichlorophen	causes allergic reactions, Ref(89)
diethanolamine see DEA	hazard: toxic, Ref(149 p.386)
diethylnitrosamine	carcinogen, Ref(16)
	carcinogenic contaminant readily passing through the skin, Ref(29)
diethylnitrosamine	carcinogen contaminant of cosmetic products, Ref(93)
digalloyl trioleate	causes photosensitivity, Ref(152,15,64)
dihydroxyacetone	causes contact allergy, Ref(194)
	causes contact allergy; adverse effects, Ref(163)
diisopropanolnitrosamine	carcinogen, Ref(16)
dimethicon	causes tumors and mutations in laboratory animals, Ref(175)
dimethyl lauramine	nitrosamines can form in all cosmetic ingredients containing amines and amino derivatives with nitrogen compounds, Ref(150); note: nitrosamines are known carcinogens, Ref(16)

Cosmetic Chemical	Reference to Adverse Reaction
dimethyl stearamine	nitrosamines can form in all cosmetic ingredients containing amines and amino derivatives with nitrogen compounds, Ref(150); note: nitrosamines are known carcinogens, Ref(16)
dioxane see also 1,4-dioxane	40% of commercial cosmetic products were shown to contain up to 85 ppm of the carcinogen 1,4-dioxane, Ref(179)
dioxybenzone (benzophenone-n (1-12))	causes contact dermatitis, Ref(117)
	causes photosensitivity, Ref(152,-25,64)
direct black 38	found to be carcinogenic, Ref(153)
direct blue 6	found to be carcinogenic, Ref(153)
disodium EDTA (ethylenediaminetetraacetic acid, disodium salt)	nitrosamines can form in all cosmetic ingredients containing amines and amino derivatives with nitrogen compounds, Ref(150); note: nitrosamines are known carcinogens, Ref(16)
disodium laureth sulfosuccinate	may contain dangerous levels of ethylen oxide and/or dioxane, both potent toxins, as a manufacturing byproduct, Ref(150)
disodium oleamido peg	may contain dangerous levels of ethylen oxide and/or dioxane, both potent toxins, as a manufacturing byproduct, Ref(150)
DMDM hydantoin	causes dermatitis, Ref(62)
Dowicil	causes allergic reactions, Ref(89)
EDTA (ethylenediaminetetraacetic acid)	nitrosamines can form in all cosmetic ingredients containing amines and amino derivatives with nitrogen compounds, Ref(150); note: nitrosamines are known carcinogens, Ref(16)
erythrosine Sodium (or potassium) salt of iodeosin; FD&C Red No,3)	cytotoxicity and genotoxicity established, Ref(63)
ethanolamine (MEA; monoethanolamine; colamine; 2-aminoethanol; 2-hydroxyethylamine)	hazard: skin irritant, Ref(149 p.474)

Cosmetic Chemical	Reference to Adverse Reaction
	nitrosamines can form in all cosmetic ingredients containing amines and amino derivatives with nitrogen compounds, Ref(150); note: nitrosamines are known carcinogens, Ref(16) & causes allergic reactions and contact dermatitis, Ref(75)
ethanolamines "Group"	causes contact dermatitis; adverse effects, Ref(26)
	causes contact dermatitis; adverse effects, Ref(55)
	causes allergic reactions and contact dermatitis; adverse effects, Ref(75)
	causes severe facial dermatitis; adverse effects, Ref(115)
ethers "Group"	causes contact dermatitis; adverse effects, Ref(61)
ethoxyethyl--methoxy cinnamate (2-ethoxyethyl-p-methoxycinnamate)	causes stinging sensations, Ref(103)
ethoxylated lanolins	has comedogenic (acne promoting) properties, Ref(82)
	may contain dangerous levels of ethylen oxide and/or dioxane, both potent toxins, as a manufacturing byproduct, Ref(150)
ethyl alcohol (alcohol, grain alcohol, ethanol)	causes systemic eczematous contact dermatitis, Ref(138)
ethyl benzoate	causes inflammatory reaction in rabbits, Ref(53)
ethyl-p-hydroxybenzoate	has low sensitizing potential, Ref(56)
ethylene glycol (ethylene alcohol; glycol, 1,2-ethanediol)	hazard: toxic by ingestion and inhalation, lethal dose reported to be 100 cc, Ref(149 p.487)
ethylene glycols "Group"	Induces allergic reactions; adverse effects, Ref(165)
	causes allergic reactions; adverse effects, Ref(166)
	has causes chemically induced contact dermatitis; adverse effects, Ref(4)

Cosmetic Chemical	Reference to Adverse Reaction
	has causes contact eczema; adverse effects, Ref(47)
ethylene oxide (epoxyethane; oxirane)	Potent toxin with NIOSH exposure limit of 1 ppm, Ref(116 p.112)
	hazard: Irritant to eyes and skin, a suspected human carcinogen, Ref(149 p.490)
ethylenediamine (1,2-diaminoethane)	hazard: toxic by inhalation and skin absorption, strong irritant to skin and eyes, Ref(149 p.485)
ethylenediamines "Group"	causes facial dermatoses and contact dermatitis; -adverse effects, Ref(39)
ethylparaben (ethyl-p-hydroxybenzoate)	causes contact dermatitis, Ref(17)
	causes allergic reactions (1,9%), Ref(89)
fatty acids	contaminated with substantial amounts of N-nitroso- N-methylalkylamines, Ref(18)
fatty alcohols "Group" (A primary alcohol from C8 to C20)	causes cosmetic allergies; adverse effects, Ref(59)
fatty amine oxides	contaminated with substantial amounts of N-nitroso-N- methylalkylamines, Ref(18)
fluorans	shown to have comedogenic (acne promoting) properties, Ref(82)
fluoranthene	carcinogen contaminant in miner oils and waxes, Ref(95)
fluoresceins "Group" (resorcinolphthalein; diresorcinolphthalein)	cytotoxicity and genotoxicity established; toxicity, Ref(63)
formaldehyde "Group"	formaldehyde released by diazolidinyl urea causes dermatitis; adverse effects, Ref(46)
	causes contact dermatitis; adverse effects, Ref(60)
	causes dermatitis; adverse effects, Ref(62)
	Induced contact dermatitis; adverse effects, Ref(65)

Cosmetic Chemical	Reference to Adverse Reaction
	causes allergic contact dermatitis; adverse effects, Ref(88)
formaldehyde (oxymethylene; formic aldehyde; methanal)	causes facial contact dermatitis, Ref(169)
	hazard: toxic by inhalation, strong irritant, a carcinogen, Ref(149 p.536)
	causes contact allergies, Ref(35)
	contaminant in shampoos and bath preparations, Ref(38)
	formaldehyde released by diazolidinyl urea causes dermatitis, Ref(46)
	formaldehyde resin derivatives causes contact dermatitis, Ref(60)
	formaldehyde contained in DMDM hydantoin causes dermatitis, Ref(61)
	causes dermatitis, Ref(62)
	formaldehyde releasers in cosmetics, Ref(84)
	donor propanediols causes allergic contact dermatitis, Ref(88)
	causes dermatitis, Ref(89)
fragrances "Group"	causes facial contact dermatitis, Ref(169)
	causes contact dermatitis, Ref(17)
furocoumarin-plus-UVA	phototoxin; reacts with UV radiation to yield genotoxin, Ref(19)
geraniol	causes pigmented contact dermatitis, Ref(40)
geranium oil	causes pigmented contact dermatitis, Ref(40)
glycerol (glycerin; glycyl alcohol; 1,2,3-propanetriol)	causes skin irritation and hypersensitivity, Ref(137)
glyceryl esters "Group"	causes contact dermatitis, Ref(129)
	causes contact dermatitis, Ref(58)
glyceryl monolaurate (glycerol monolaurate)	causes irritation, Ref(58)

Cosmetic Chemical	Reference to Adverse Reaction
glyceryl monostearate (glycerol monostearate, monostearin)	causes skin allergy, Ref(58)
glyceryl oleate	causes skin allergies, Ref(129)
glyceryl PABA	causes photosensitivity, Ref(152, 25,64)
glyceryl stearate	causes skin allergy, Ref(58)
glyceryl thioglycolate	causes allergic contact dermatitis, Ref(181)
	causes allergic contact dermatitis (eczematous dermatitis of both hands), Ref(3)
glycols "Group" (see ethylene glycol; general term for dihydric alcohols which are physically and chemically similar to glycerol)	causes delayed contact allergy; adverse effects, Ref(41)
grain alcohol (ethyl alcohol, ethanol)	causes systemic eczematous contact dermatitis, Ref(138)
hexachlorophene	system toxin in infants, Ref(111)
	hazard: FDA prohibits use unless prescribed by a physician, Ref(149 p.597)
hexamidine diisethionate	causes facial dermatoses and contact dermatitis, Ref(39)
hexylene glycol (4-methyl-2,4-pentanediol)	hazard: toxic by ingestion and inhalation; irritant to skin, eyes, and mucous membranes, Ref(149 p.602)
	causes delayed contact allergy, Ref(41)
homesalate (homomenthyl salicylate)	causes follicular eruption, Ref(152, 25,64)
hydantoins "Group" (glycolylurea)	causes dermatitis; adverse effects, Ref(62)
hydrocarbons "Group"	causes chemically induced acne, (Ref(17)
	causes chemically induced acne, Ref(82)
	causes chemically induced acne, Ref(120)

Cosmetic Chemical	Reference to Adverse Reaction
	contains carcinogen contaminant, Ref(95)
	contain carcinogen contaminant, Ref(197)
hydrogen peroxide	tumor and cancer causes agent; Ref(175)
hydroquinone (quinol; hydroquinol; p-dohydroxybenzene)	causes hyperpigmentation (brown globules), Ref(182)
	hazard: toxic by ingestion and inhalation, irritant, Ref(149 p.619)
	causes severe skin damage, Ref(9)
hydroquinones "Group"	causes exogenous ochronosis, a hyperpigmentation of the face; adverse effects, Ref(156)
	causes allergic contact dermatitis; adverse effects, Ref(74)
	causes allergic contact dermatitis; adverse effects, Ref(80)
	causes contact dermatitis; adverse effects, Ref(94)
hydroxy citronellal	causes facial psoriasis; adverse effects, Ref(86)
hydroxy propylmethyl cellulose	mild eye and skin irritant, Ref(183)
hydroxybenzoic acids	causes contact dermatitis; adverse effects, Ref(13)
hydroxycitronella (citronellal hydrate; 3,7-dimethyl-7- hydroxyoctenal)	causes allergies and contact dermatitis (in perfume ingredient), Ref(30)
	causes pigmented contact dermatitis, Ref(40)
	causes facial psoriasis, Ref(86)
hydroxycoumarins	found to be a skin sensitizer, Ref(42)
hydroxypropyl aminobenzoate	nitrosamines can form in all cosmetic ingredients containing amines and amino derivatives with nitrogen compounds, Ref(150); note: nitrosamines are known carcinogens, Ref(16)

Cosmetic Chemical	Reference to Adverse Reaction
hydroxypropylcellulose	mild irritant, Ref(159)
imidazolidinyl urea	causes dermatitis, Ref(64)
indigoids	shown to have comedogenic (acne promoting) properties, Ref(82)
isoceteth-n	may contain dangerous levels of ethylen oxide and dioxane, both potent toxins, as a manufacturing byproduct, Ref(150)
isocetyl stearate (isocetyl laurate)	shown to have comedogenic (acne promoting) properties, Ref(82)
isoeugenol	causes contact dermatitis, Ref(23)
isolaureth-n	may contain dangerous levels of ethylen oxide and dioxane, both potent toxins, as a manufacturing byproduct, Ref(150)
isopropyl isostearate	has comedogenic (acne promoting) properties, Ref(82)
	has comedogenic (acne promoting) properties, Ref(82)
isopropyl palmitate	causes skin irritation and dermatitis in rabbits, Ref(79)
	shown to have comedogenic (acne promoting) properties, Ref(82)
isopropyl-hydroxypalmityl-ether	causes contact allergies, Ref(61)
isopropylmyristate	has comedogenic (acne promoting) properties, Ref(82)
isopropylmyristate (and its analogs)	shown to have comedogenic (acne promoting) properties, Ref(82)
isopsoralen	causes cutaneous phototoxicity reactions, Ref(66)
isostearamide DEA	nitrosamines can form in all cosmetic ingredients containing amines and amino derivatives with nitrogen compounds, Ref(150); note: nitrosamines are known carcinogens, Ref(16)
isosteareth-n	may contain dangerous levels of ethylen oxide and dioxane, both potent toxins, as a manufacturing byproduct, Ref(150)

Cosmetic Chemical	Reference to Adverse Reaction
isostearyl neopentanoate	has comedogenic (acne promoting) properties, Ref(82)
	shown to have comedogenic (acne promoting) properties, Ref(82)
isothiazolinone	has causes contact dermatitis, Ref(21)
ivy extract	causes irritant and allergic dermatitis, Ref(120)
kohl	Caution! causes lead and antimony poisoning, Ref(184)
lanolin	causes contact dermatitis, Ref(17)
lanolin "Group"	has comedogenic (acne promoting) properties; toxicity, Ref(82)
lanolin alcohol	shown to have comedogenic (acne promoting) properties, Ref(120 9-2)
lanolin and lanolin derivatives	causes adverse skin reactions, Ref(196)
lanolin, acetylated	causes contact dermatitis, Ref(17)
	shown to have comedogenic (acne promoting) properties, Ref(82)
lanolin, ethoxylated	causes contact dermatitis, Ref(17)
	shown to have comedogenic (acne promoting) properties, Ref(82)
lauramide dea	nitrosamines can form in all cosmetic ingredients containing amines and amino derivatives with nitrogen compounds, Ref(150); note: nitrosamines are known carcinogens, Ref(16)
lauramidopropyl dimethylamine	causes contact allergic reactions, Ref(45)
laurel oil	causes severe allergies, Ref(67)
laureth-n	may contain dangerous levels of ethylene oxide and/or dioxane, both potent toxins, as a manufacturing byproduct, Ref(150)
lauryl alcohol (alcohol C12; n-dodecanol; dodecyl alcohol)	has acneigenic properties, Ref(130)
lavender oil	causes contact allergies and photo sensitivity, Ref(128)

Cosmetic Chemical	Reference to Adverse Reaction
lemon extract	juice causes dermatitis, Ref(120)
lemon oil (lemon peel oil)	causes photo toxicity, Ref(120)
	causes pigmented contact dermatitis, Ref(40)
lemon peel	causes dermatitis, Ref(120)
linalool (linalol, 3,7-dimethyl-1,6-octadien-3-ol)	causes facial psoriasis; adverse effects, Ref(86)
	causes facial psoriasis, Ref(86)
lineoleamide dea	nitrosamines can form in all cosmetic ingredients containing amines and amino derivatives with nitrogen compounds, Ref(150); note: nitrosamines are known carcinogens, Ref(16)
linoleamidopropyl ethly dimonium ethosulfate	nitrosamines can form in all cosmetic ingredients containing amines and amino derivatives with nitrogen compounds, Ref(150); note: nitrosamines are known carcinogens, Ref(16)
linseed oil (flaxseed oil)	shown to promote acne, Ref(72)
m-phenylenediamine (m-diaminobenzene)	found to be mutagenic, Ref(154)
	shows mutagenic properties, Ref(101)
m-toluenediamine (mTD; toluene-2,4-diamine)	shows decisive mutagenicity both on the X-chromosome and the RNA genes of the human male, Ref(106)
	hazard: a carcinogen, Ref(149, p.1163)
magnesium laureth sulfate	may contain dangerous levels of ethylen oxide ethylen oxide and/or dioxane, both potent toxins, as a manufacturing byproduct, Ref(150)
magnesium oleth sulfate	may contain dangerous levels of ethylen oxide and/or dioxane, both potent toxins, as a manufacturing byproduct, Ref(150)
mercuric chloride, ammoniated (Mercury, ammoniated)	hazard: highly toxic, Ref(149 p.746)

Cosmetic Chemical	Reference to Adverse Reaction
mercuric ammonium chloride	Poses considerable health risk, systemic poison, Ref(25)
mercuric chloride "Group"	causes nephrotic syndrome; adverse effects , Ref(23)
mercuric chloride (mercury bichloride; mercury chloride)	hazard: toxic by ingestion, inhalation, and skin absorption; a poison, Ref(149 p.742)
mercury chloride, ammoniated	causes dermatitis, Ref(89)
metals "Group"	causes contact dermatitis on hands, Ref(170)
methaninie (quaternium 15)	causes induced contact dermatitis, Ref(28)
methenamine "Group" (hexamethylenetetramine; methenamine; HMTA; aminoform)	hazard: skin irritant, flammable, dangerous fire risk, Ref(149 p.600)
	causes contact dermatitis; adverse effects, Ref(65)
methoxsalen (5-methoxypsoralen)	causes burns by photosensitation, Ref(185)
	causes burns by photosensitization, Ref(171)
methyl alcohol "Group" (methanol; wood alcohol)	causes contact eczema; adverse effects, Ref(100)
	hazard: toxic by ingestion (causes blindness), Ref(149 p.757)
methyl benzoate (benzoic acid, methyl ester; niobe oil)	hazard: toxic by ingestion, Ref(149 p.760)
	causes inflammatory reaction in rabbits, Ref(53)
methyl chloroisothiazolinine	causes cosmetic allergies, Ref(50)
methyl gluceth	may contain dangerous levels of dioxane, both potent toxins, as a manufacturing byproduct, Ref(150)
methyl glucose sesquisterarate	causes dermatitis, Ref(78)
methyl glucoside (methyl-alpha-d-glycopyranoside)	causes dermatitis, Ref(78)

Cosmetic Chemical	Reference to Adverse Reaction
methyl methacrylate	hazard: Flammable, dangerous fire risk, explosive limits in air 2,1-12,5%, Ref(149 p.774)
methyl methacrylates "Group"	causes adverse nail reactions; adverse effects, Ref(32)
	causes contact dermatitis; adverse effects, Ref(99)
methyl oleate	has acneigenic properties, Ref(130)
methylcellulose, see hydroxy propylmethyl cellulose	mild eye and skin irritant, Ref(183)
methylchloroisothiazolinone	causes cosmetic allergies, Ref(50)
methyldibromo glutaronitrile (Tektamer 38)	causes allergic contact dermatitis, Ref(180)
	causes allergic reactions, Ref(177)
	causes allergic reactions, Ref(186)
	causes allergic reactions, Ref(166)
methylisothiazolinine	causes cosmetic allergies, Ref(50)
	has causes cosmetic allergies, Ref(50)
methylparaben (methyl-p-hydroxybenzoate)	shown to have low sensitizing potential, Ref(56)
	hazard: toxic, Use in foods restricted to 0.1%, Ref(149 p.777)
mineral oil	causes discoloration of skin and appendages, Ref(131)
	contains polycyclic aromatic hydrocarbons (PAH) which is mutagenic, and the carcinogen anthanthrene, Ref(95)
	has acneigenic properties, Ref(130)
MIPA (monoisopropanolamine; isopropanolamine)	causes severe eye and skin irritations, Ref(175)

Cosmetic Chemical	Reference to Adverse Reaction
	nitrosamines can form in all cosmetic ingredients containing amines and amino derivatives with nitrogen compounds, ref(150); note: nitrosamines are known carcinogens, Ref(16)
	causes allergic reactions and contact dermatitis, Ref(75)
modulan	has causes skin irritation and histological changes in rabbits, Ref(79)
monoazoanilies	shown to have comedogenic (acne promoting) properties, Ref(82)
monoethanolamine sulfite	causes allergic reactions and contact dermatitis, Ref(75)
	nitrosamines can form in all cosmetic ingredients containing amines and amino derivatives with nitrogen compounds, Ref(150); note: nitrosamines are known carcinogens, Ref(16)
monotertiary butyl hydroquinone	causes contact dermatitis, Ref(94)
	causes allergic contact dermatitis, Ref(80)
moskene	causes pigmented contact dermatitis, Ref(187)
musk ambrette	causes pigmented photoallergic contact dermatitis, Ref(12)
musk moskene	causes pigmented contact dermatitis and hyperpigmentation, Ref(167)
myristamidopropyl dimethylamine	causes contact allergic reactions, Ref(45)
myristates "Group"	shown to have comedogenic (acne promoting) properties; toxicity, Ref(82)
myristyl alcohol (1-tetradecanol)	causes cosmetic allergies, Ref(59)
myristyl myristate	has comedogenic (acne promoting) properties, Ref(82)
myristyl propionate	has comedogenic (acne promoting) properties, Ref(82)

Cosmetic Chemical	Reference to Adverse Reaction
n-butyl benzoate (butyl benzoate)	causes inflammatory reaction in rabbits, Ref(53)
n-nitroso compounds	carcinogen contaminant in cosmetic products, Ref(77)
n-nitroso-n-methylalkylamines	carcinogen contaminant of fatty amine oxides, Ref(18)
n-nitroso-n-methyltetradecyl amine	carcinogen contaminant of fatty amine oxides, Ref(18)
n-nitrosoalkanolamines	carcinogen, Ref(16)
n-nitrosobis(2-hydroxypropyl)amine	carcinogen, Ref(16)
n-nitrosodiethanolamine (dimethylnitrosamine)	carcinogen contaminant in cosmetic products, Ref(77)
	carcinogen, Ref(16)
	carcinogenic contaminant readily passing through the skin, Ref(29)
	carcinogen contaminant of cosmetic products, Ref(93)
	hazard: a carcinogen, Ref(149 p.832)
n-nitrosodimethylamine	carcinogen contaminant in cosmetic products, Ref(77)
n-nitrosomorpholine	carcinogen contaminant in cosmetic products, Ref(77)
n-propyl benzoate	causes inflammatory reaction in rabbits, Ref(53)
n-propylamines	hazard: strong irritant to skin and tissue, Ref(149 p.972)
naphthalene, (tar camphor)	hazard: toxic by inhalation, Ref(149 p.806)
naphthalenes "Group" (tar camphor)	can produce hyperirretability and other system effects; toxicity, Ref(98)
naphthoquinone	hazard: Irritant, Ref(149 p.808)
naphtol	causes severe eye and skin irritation; Ref(175)
naphtoquinones "Group"	causes contact dermatitis; adverse effects, Ref(27)

Cosmetic Chemical	Reference to Adverse Reaction
neomycin	causes contact dermatitis, Ref(17)
nickel	causes contact dermatitis, Ref(17)
	hazard: a carcinogen (OSHA), Ref(149 p.819)
	causes eyelid dermatitis (found in eyelash curler), Ref(7)
	causes contact allergies, Ref(33)
	causes contact eczema, Ref(47)
nickle sulfate	causes facial contact dermatitis, Ref(169)
nitriles "Group"	causes allergic reactions; adverse effects, Ref(165)
	causes allergic reactions; adverse effects, Ref(166)
	causes contact eczema; adverse effects, Ref(47)
	causes chemically induced contact dermatitis; adverse effects , Ref(4)
nitrilotriacetic acid	found to be carcinogenic, Ref(153)
nitrobenzene (oil of mirbane)	hazard: toxic by ingestion, inhalation, and skin absorption, Ref(149 p.825)
nitrobenzenes "Group"	carcinogen contaminant of cosmetic products; adverse effects, Ref(93)
nitrosamines	cancer-causes cosmetic contaminant and carcinogens, Ref(16)
nonylphenol	causes skin irritation and dermatitis in rabbits, Ref(79)
novocain (TM for a brand of procaine hydrochloride)	causes dermatitis, Ref(70)
o-nitro-p-aminophenol	found to be carcinogenic, Ref(153)
o-phenylenediamine	found to be carcinogenic, Ref(153)
	found to be mutagenic, Ref(154)
oak moss	causes allergies and skin irritations, Ref(120 p.297)
	Contact dermatitis, Ref(23)

Cosmetic Chemical	Reference to Adverse Reaction
octyl palmitate	shown to have comedogenic (acne promoting) properties, Ref(82)
octyl palmitate	shown to have comedogenic (acne promoting) properties, Ref(82)
octyl stearate	shown to have comedogenic (acne promoting) properties, Ref(82)
octyoxynol-n	may contain dangerous levels of ethylen oxide and/or dioxane, both potent toxins, as a manufacturing byproduct, Ref(150)
oil of purcellin	causes skin irritation and dermatitis in rabbits, Ref(79)
oleamidopropyl dimethylamine	has causes contact allergic reactions, Ref(45)
	causes contact dermatitis demonstrated, Ref(73)
oleic acid (cis-9-octadecenoic acid; red oil)	has acneigenic properties, Ref(130)
oleth-n	may contain dangerous levels of ethylen oxide and/or dioxane, both potent toxins, as a manufacturing byproduct, Ref(150)
olive oil	has acneigenic properties, Ref(130)
oxybenzone	causes contact dermatitis, Ref(176)
p-aminobenzoic acid	causes photo sensitivity and contact dermatitis, Ref(120)
p-phenylenediamine (p-diaminobenzene)	shows mutagenic activity in metabolically active germ cells (spermatids and spermatocytes), Ref(107)
	hazard: toxic by ingestion and inhalation, strong irritant to skin, Ref(149 p.902)
PABA (p-aminobenzoic acid)	causes photo sensitivity and contact dermatitis, Ref(120)
palmitates "Group"	causes contact dermatitis; adverse effects, Ref(61)
palmitic acids "Group" (hexadecanoic acid; cetylic acid)	causes contact dermatitis; adverse effects, Ref(61)
parabens	causes allergic reactions, Ref(89)

Cosmetic Chemical	Reference to Adverse Reaction
parabens (TM for the methyl, propyl, butyl, and ethyl esters of p-hydroxybenzoic acid)	causes dermatitis, Ref(17)
paraffin	may contain benzo-a-pyrene and benzo-b-fluroanthene, two well known carcinogens, Ref(197)
	possible carcinogen contaminant; polycyclic aromatic hydrocarbons (PAH), Ref(95)
paraphenylenediamine	causes contact dermatitis, Ref(30)
paraphenylenediamine dihydrochloride	causes facial contact dermatitis, Ref(169)
parsley seed oil	causes irritant and allergic dermatitis, Ref(120)
PEG (Abbreviation for polyethylene glycol; polyoxethylene; polyglycol; polyether glycol)	may contain dangerous levels of dioxane, a potent toxins, as a manufacturing byproduct, Ref(150)
peg-n stearate	may contain dangerous levels of dioxane, a potent toxins, as a manufacturing byproduct, Ref(150)
peg-n (4-200)	may contain dangerous levels of dioxane, a potent toxin, as a manufacturing byproduct, Ref(150)
peppermint oil	causes irritant and allergic dermatitis, Ref(120)
perfume "Group"	causes pigmented contact dermatitis and hyperpigmentation; adverse effects, Ref(167)
persulphates, alkaline	causes asthma in hair dressers, Ref(102)
perylene	carcinogen contaminant in mineral oils and waxes, Ref(95)
petrolatum	causes discoloration of skin and appendages, Ref(131)
	may contain benzo-a-pyrene and benzo-b-fluroanthene, two well known carcinogens, Ref(197)

Cosmetic Chemical	Reference to Adverse Reaction
	possible carcinogen contaminant; polycyclic aromatic hydrocarbons (PAH), Ref(95)
phenacetin, (USP name for acetophenetidin; p-acetylphenetidin; acetophenetidide; p-ethoxyacetanilide)	mutagenic and carcinogenic properties, Ref(91)
	hazard: toxic by ingestion, Ref(149 p.9)
phenoxyethanol	causes allergic reactions, Ref(177)
	causes allergic reactions, Ref(186)
phenylenediamines "Group"	causes facial contact dermatitis; adverse effects, Ref(169)
	mutagenic activity in metabolically active germ cells (spermatids and spermatocytes); toxicity, Ref(107)
phthalates "Group"	mutagenic, cancerogenic and orchidotoxic properties, Ref(22)
phthalic acids "Group" (o-phthalic acid; o-benzene dicarboxylic acid)	mutagenic, cancerogenic and orchidotoxic properties, Ref(22)
pinene	causes contact dermatitis, Ref(76)
polycyclic aromatic hydrocarbons (PAH)	carcinogen contaminant of mineral oil products, Ref(95)
polyethoxylated compounds	48% of cosmetic products containing polyethoxylated surfactants were found to contain 7.3 - 85.9 ppm of 1,4-dioxane, Ref(162)
polyoxyethylene sorbitan monooleate	causes contact dermatitis, Ref(26)
	causes contact dermatitis, Ref(26)
polypropylene glycole	causes skin irritation and dermatitis; adverse effects, Ref(90)
polysorbate-n (20-85)	causes contact sensitivity and irritation, Ref(134)
potassium hydroxide	causes severe eye and skin irritation, Ref(175)
PPG, see polypropylene glycole	causes skin irritation and dermatitis; adverse effects, Ref(90)

Cosmetic Chemical	Reference to Adverse Reaction
PPG-2-isodeceth-4	may contain dangerous levels of ethylen oxide and/or dioxane, both potent toxins, as a manufacturing byproduct, Ref(150)
PPG-m ceteth-n	may contain dangerous levels of ethylen oxide and/or dioxane, both potent toxins, as a manufacturing byproduct, Ref(150)
procaine "Group"	In cream causes dermatitis; toxicity, Ref(70)
procaine hydrochloride (procaine)	causes systemic eczematous contact-type dermatitis, Ref(129)
propanediols "Group"	causes delayed contact allergy; adverse effects, Ref(41)
	causes skin irritation and dermatitis; adverse effects, Ref(90)
	causes unilateral mydriasis; adverse effects, Ref(109)
propantheline bromide	causes unilateral mydriasis, Ref(109)
propolis (beeswax)	causes hypersensitivity and irritation, Ref(133)
propyl gallate	causes contact allergies, Ref(49)
	hazard: Use in foods restricted to 0.02% of fat content, Ref(149 p.974)
propylamines "Group"	causes contact allergic reactions; adverse effects, Ref(45)
	causes contact dermatitis demonstrated; adverse effects, Ref(73)
propylene glycol	causes delayed contact allergy, Ref(41)
	causes skin irritation and dermatitis, Ref(90)
	has comedogenic (acne promoting) properties, Ref(82)
	causes skin irritation and dermatitis; adverse effects, Ref(90)
	causes contact dermatitis, Ref(195)
	causes contact dermatitis, Ref(196)

Cosmetic Chemical	Reference to Adverse Reaction
propylene glycol ceteth-n	may contain dangerous levels of dioxane, a potent toxins, as a manufacturing byproduct, Ref(150)
propylene glycol-2 myristyl propionate	shown to have comedogenic (acne promoting) properties, Ref(82)
propylparaben (propyl-p-hydroxybenzoate)	causes dermatitis, Ref(17)
	shown to have low sensitizing potential, Ref(56)
	causes allergic reactions (1,9%), Ref(89)
psoralen (furocoumarines)	phototoxin; reacts with UV radiation to yield genotoxin, Ref(19)
psoralens "Group"	causes cutaneous phototoxicity reactions; adverse effects, Ref(66)
purcellin, oil of	has causes skin irritation and histological changes in rabbits, Ref(79)
quaternium-15	induced contact dermatitis, Ref(28)
	induced contact dermatitis, Ref(65)
quaternium-n (quaternary ammonium compounds)	caused fatal drug allergy (anaphylactic shock), Ref(189)
	may cause increased sensitivity to muscle relaxant (anaphylactic shock), Ref(190)
	causes contact dermatitis, Ref(65)
quinaldine (chinaldine; alpha-methylquinoline)	hazard: strong irritant to mucous membranes, Ref(149 p.990)
quinaldines "Group" (chinaldine; alpha-methylquinoline)	causes dermatitis; adverse effects, Ref(92)
	causes dermatitis; adverse effects, Ref(105)
quinazoline yellow	causes dermatitis, Ref(92)
quinoline yellow	causes allergic contact dermatitis, Ref(83)
quinolines "Group" (chinoline)	causes allergic contact dermatitis; adverse effects, Ref(83)

Cosmetic Chemical	Reference to Adverse Reaction
	causes dermatitis; adverse effects, Ref(105)
quinophthalone (Yellow No, 33)	causes dermatitis, Ref(105)
red dyes "Group"	all D&C red dyes tested to date are shown to have comedogenic (acne promoting) properties; toxicity, Ref(82)
red no. 3	Cytotoxicity and genotoxicity established, Ref(63)
red no. 36	causes dermatitis, Ref(69)
red no. 40	carcinogen amine contamination found, Ref(43)
red petrolatum (see also petrolatum)	causes discoloration of skin and appendages, Ref(131)
resins "Group"	causes contact dermatitis on hands, Ref(170)
	causes eyelid dermatitis; adverse effects, Ref(172)
	causes allergic reactions; adverse effects, Ref(54)
Rhodamine B	decreasing collagen content on the fibroblast cell layer of the human lip. Can impair the formation on extracellular matrix which is important for the maintenance of the lip tissue, Ref(155)
	can inhibit skin cell metabolism, Ref(2)
Rhodamines "Group"	can inhibit skin cell metabolism; adverse effects, Ref(2)
ricinoleamidopropyl dimethylamine lactate	causes contact allergic reactions, Ref(45)
ricinoleic acid	causes dermatitis, Ref(85)
rosemary extract	causes irritancy and allergic dermatitis, photosensitivity, Ref(120)
rosin	causes allergic reactions, Ref(54)
scoparone	found to be a skin sensitizer, Ref(42)
secondary amines	recommended not to be used in Europe, Ref(16)

Cosmetic Chemical	Reference to Adverse Reaction
sesquiterpene "Group"	causes severe allergies; adverse effects, Ref(67)
sesquiterpene lactone	causes severe allergies (laurel allergy), Ref(67)
silica (silicon dioxide)	hazard: toxic by inhalation, chronic exposure to dust may cause silicosis, Ref(149 p.1038)
	delayed hypersensitivity reaction, Ref(51)
silk	causes contact urticaria, Ref(139)
sodium benzoate	causes allergic reactions, Ref(89)
	hazard: Use in foods limited to 0.1%, Ref(149 p.1053)
sodium dodecyl sulfate	causes contact eczema, Ref(100)
sodium hydroxide	causes severe skin and eye irritation, Ref(175)
sodium laureth-n sulfate	causes skin irritation and dermatitis, Ref(132)
	may contain dangerous levels of ethylen oxide and/or dioxane, both potent toxins, as a manufacturing byproduct, Ref(150)
sodium lauryl sulfate	causes contact eczema, Ref(100)
sodium oleth sulfate	may contain dangerous levels of ethylen oxide and/or dioxane, both potent toxins, as a manufacturing byproduct, Ref(150)
sodium trideceth sulfate	may contain dangerous levels of ethylen oxide and/or dioxane, both potent toxins, as a manufacturing byproduct, Ref(150)
sorbic acid (2,4-hexadienoic acid)	causes contact urticaria, Ref(126)
sorbitan laurate	causes contact urticaria, Ref(126)
sorbitan oleate	causes contact urticaria, Ref(126)
sorbitan palmitate	causes contact dermatitis, Ref(26)
sorbitan sequioleate	causes contact dermatitis, Ref(26)
sorbitan stearate	causes contact urticaria Ref(126)
stearamidoethyl diethylamine phosphate	causes allergic contact dermatitis, Ref(81)

Cosmetic Chemical	Reference to Adverse Reaction
stearamidopropyl dimethylamine	secondary amines causes allergic dermatitis and have carcinogen properties, Ref(81)
stearamin oxyd	nitrosamines can form in all cosmetic ingredients containing amines and amino derivatives with nitrogen compounds, Ref(150); note: nitrosamines are known carcinogens, Ref(16)
steareth-n	may contain -dangerous levels of ethylen oxide and/or dioxane, both potent toxins, as a manufacturing byproduct, Ref(150)
stearic acid (n-octadecanoic acid)	causes skin allergy, Ref(58)
stearic acids "Group"	causes dermatitis; adverse effects, Ref(78)
stearic acids "Group"	causes allergic contact dermatitis; adverse effects, Ref(81)
stearyl alcohol (1-octadecanol; octadecyl alcohol)	causes contact dermatitis and allergies, Ref(135, 136)
sulisobenzone (benzophenone-4)	causes photosensitivity, Ref(152, 25,64)
talc (talcum; soapstone; steatite)	hazard: toxic by inhalation, Ref(149 p.1117)
	some talc found to contain amphibole particle distribution typical of asbestos (which is cancer causes), Ref(1)
tallow amidopropyl dimethylamine	has causes contact allergic reactions, Ref(45)
TEA (Abbreviation for triethanolamine)	nitrosamines can form in all cosmetic ingredients containing amines and amino derivatives with nitrogen compounds, Ref(150); note: nitrosamines are known carcinogens, Ref(16)
TEA carbomer	triethanolamine compounds causes severe facial dermatitis, Ref(115)

Cosmetic Chemical	Reference to Adverse Reaction
	nitrosamines can form in all cosmetic ingredients containing amines and amino derivatives with nitrogen compounds, Ref(150); note: nitrosamines are known carcinogens, Ref(16)
TEA coco hydrolyzed protein	causes severe facial dermatitis, Ref(115)
TEA cocoyl glutamate	triethanolamine compounds causes severe facial dermatitis, Ref(115)
	nitrosamines can form in all cosmetic ingredients containing amines and amino derivatives with nitrogen compounds, Ref(150); note: nitrosamines are known carcinogens, Ref(16)
TEA lauryl sulfate	nitrosamines can form in all cosmetic ingredients containing amines and amino derivatives with nitrogen compounds, Ref(150); note: nitrosamines are known carcinogens, Ref(16)
TEA salicylate	can form cancer causes nitrosoamines in sunlight (phototoxin), Ref(150)
TEA stearate (trihydroxyethylamine stearate)	triethanolamine compounds causes severe facial dermatitis, Ref(115)
	nitrosamines can form in all cosmetic ingredients containing amines and amino derivatives with nitrogen compounds, Ref(150); note: nitrosamines are known carcinogens, Ref(16)
TEA-Coco hydrolyzed protein	triethanolamine compounds causes severe facial dermatitis, Ref(115)
	nitrosamines can form in all cosmetic ingredients containing amines and amino derivatives with nitrogen compounds, Ref(150); note: nitrosamines are known carcinogens, Ref(16); triethanolamine compounds causes severe facial dermatitis, Ref(115)
terpenes "Group"	causes facial psoriasis; adverse effects, Ref(86)

Cosmetic Chemical	Reference to Adverse Reaction
turpentine oil	causes contact dermatitis, Ref(76)
tertiary ammonium compounds	caused fatal drug allergy (anaphylactic shock), Ref(189)
	may cause increased sensitivity to muscle relaxant (anaphylactic shock), Ref(190)
	causes contact dermatitis, Ref(65)
tetrahydronaphthalene	hazard: irritant to eyes and skin, Ref(149 p.1136)
tetrahydronaphthalenes "Group"	can produce hyperirritability and other system effects, Ref(98)
tetrasodium EDTA (ethylenediaminetetraacetic acid, tetrasodium salt)	nitrosamines can form in all cosmetic ingredients containing amines and amino derivatives with nitrogen compounds, Ref(150); note: nitrosamines are known carcinogens, Ref(16)
thiazoles "Group"	causes allergic reactions; adverse effects, Ref(165)
	are mutagens and produce contact allergy and dermatitis; adverse effects, Ref(6)
	has caused contact dermatitis; adverse effects, Ref(21)
	causes contact allergies; adverse effects, Ref(33)
	causes cosmetic allergies; adverse effects, Ref(50)
thioglycolates, (see glyceryl or ammonium thioglycolate)	
thiomersal	causes dermatitis, Ref(17)
thyme extract	causes contact allergy, Ref(120)
tocopherol (vitamin E)	causes contact dermatitis, Ref(127)
toluenesulfonamide formaldehyde resin	causes contact dermatitis, Ref(60)
triethanolamine (TEA)	causes contact dermatitis, Ref(26)
	causes contact dermatitis, Ref(55)

Cosmetic Chemical	Reference to Adverse Reaction
	causes severe facial dermatitis, Ref(115)
	nitrosamines can form in all cosmetic ingredients containing amines and amino derivatives with nitrogen compounds, Ref(150); nitrosamines are known carcinogens, Ref(16)
triethanolamine salts	triethanolamine causes severe facial dermatitis, Ref(115)
ultraviolet (UV) rays	hazard: dangerous to eyes, overexposure causes severe skin burns (sunburn), Ref(149 p.1204)
urea	can impair functions of the skin, cause thinning of the epidermis, and exert changes in the skin in high concentrations, Ref(110)
urea "Group" (carbamide)	causes contact dermatitis; adverse effects, Ref(34)
	causes dermatitis; adverse effects, Ref(46)
	causes dermatitis; adverse effects, Ref(64)
	induced contact dermatitis; adverse effects, Ref(65)
urocanic acid	phototoxin, Ref(160)
valerates "Group"	causes contact dermatitis and is a suspect carcinogen; adverse effects, Ref(68)
witch hazel extract	causes allergic contact dermatitis, Ref(120)
wood alcohol (methyl alcohol)	causes facial contact dermatitis, Ref(169)
	systemic poison, mutagenic effects in animals, Ref(175)
xanthene (dibenzopyran, tricyclic)	inhibits cell metabolism, Ref(193)
	shown to have comedogenic (acne promoting) properties, Ref(82)

Cosmetic Chemical	Reference to Adverse Reaction
yellow No. 11	causes allergic contact dermatitis, Ref(83)
	causes dermatitis, Ref(92)

Appendix B Colorants Approved by the FDA

Table B-1 Colors Approved by the FDA

Colorant	Remarks
Aluminum powder	External use only. May also be used in cosmetics intended for use in the area of the eye, Ref(217).
Annatto	May also be used in cosmetics intended for use in the area of the eye, Ref(217).
Beta-Carotene	May also be used in cosmetics intended for use in the area of the eye, Ref(217).
Bismuth citrate	Hair dyes for scalp only; 0.5% max. Ref(217).
Bismuth oxychloride	May also be used in cosmetics intended for use in the area of the eye, Ref(217).
Bronze powder	May also be used in cosmetics intended for use in the area of the eye, Ref(217).
Caramel	May also be used in cosmetics intended for use in the area of the eye, Ref(217).
Carmine	May also be used in cosmetics intended for use in the area of the eye, Ref(217).
Chromium hydroxide green	External use only. May also be used in cosmetics intended for use in the area of the eye, Ref(217).
Chromium oxide greens	External use only. May also be used in cosmetics intended for use in the area of the eye, Ref(217).
Copper powder	May also be used in cosmetics intended for use in the area of the eye, Ref(217).
D&C Blue No. 4	External use only, Ref(217).
D&C Brown No. 1	External use only, Ref(217).
D&C Green No. 5	No reports on adverse effects.
D&C Green No. 6	External use only, Ref(217).
D&C Green No. 8	External use only. 0.01% max., Ref(217).
D&C Orange No. 10	External use only, Ref(217).
D&C Orange No. 11	External use only, Ref(217).

Colorant	Remarks
D&C Orange No. 4	5.0% max. in lipstick and other lip cosmetics; ingested mouthwashes and dentifrices; externally applied cosmetics. Ref(217).
D&C Orange No. 5	External use only, Ref(217).
D&C Red No. 17	Shown to have acne promoting properties, Ref(82). External use only, Ref(217).
D&C Red No. 21	Shown to have acne promoting properties, Ref(82).
D&C Red No. 22	Shown to have acne promoting properties, Ref(82).
D&C Red No. 27	Shown to have acne promoting properties, Ref(82).
D&C Red No. 28	Shown to have acne promoting properties, Ref(82).
D&C Red No. 30	Shown to have acne promoting properties, Ref(82).
D&C Red No. 31	Shown to have acne promoting properties, Ref(82). External use only, Ref(217).
D&C Red No. 33	Shown to have acne promoting properties, Ref(82). Cosmetic lip products only; 3% max. Mouthwashes, dentifrices and externally applied cosmetics only, Ref(217).
D&C Red No. 34	Shown to have acne promoting properties, Ref(82). External use only, Ref(217).
D&C Red No. 36	Causes dermatitis, Ref(69). Shown to have acne promoting properties, Ref(82). Cosmetic lip products only; 3% max. Externally applied cosmetics only, Ref(217).
D&C Red No. 6	Shown to have acne promoting properties, Ref(82).
D&C Red No. 7	Shown to have acne promoting properties, Ref(82).
D&C Violet No. 2	External use only, Ref(217).
D&C Yellow No. 10	No reports on adverse effects.
D&C Yellow No. 11	Causes allergic contact dermatitis, Ref(83). Causes dermatitis, Ref(92). External use only, Ref(217).
D&C Yellow No. 7	External use only, Ref(217).
D&C Yellow No. 8	External use only, Ref(217).
Dihydroxacetone	Externally applied cosmetics intended solely or in part for imparting color to the human body only, Ref(217).
Disodium EDTA-copper	EDTA can form nitrosamines (a known carcinogen), Ref(150). Shampoos only, Ref(217).

Colorant	Remarks
Ext. D&C Violet No. 2	External use only, Ref(217).
Ext. D&C Yellow No. 7	External use only, Ref(217).
FD&C Blue No. 1	No reports on adverse effects.
FD&C Green No. 3	No reports on adverse effects.
FD&C Red No. 4	External use only, Ref(217).
FD&C Red No. 40	Ammine contamination found, Ref(43).
FD&C Yellow No. 5	No reports on adverse effects.
FD&C Yellow No. 6	No reports on adverse effects.
Ferric ammonium ferrocyanide	External use only. May also be used in cosmetics intended for use in the area of the eye, Ref(217).
Ferric ferrocyanide	External use only. May also be used in cosmetics intended for use in the area of the eye, Ref(217).
Guaiazulene	External use only, Ref(217).
Guanine	May also be used in cosmetics intended for use in the area of the eye, Ref(217).
Henna	Hair dyes only, not near eye, Ref(271).
Lead acetate	Hair dyes for scalp only; 0.6% max. as Lead, Ref(217).
Manganese violet	May also be used in cosmetics intended for use in the area of the eye, Ref(217).
Mica	May also be used in cosmetics intended for use in the area of the eye, Ref(217).
Potassium sodium copper chlorophyllin	Dentifrices only; 0.1% max, Ref(217).
Pyrophyllite	External use only, Ref(217).
Silver	Fingernail polish only; 1% max.
Synthetic iron oxides	May also be used in cosmetics intended for use in the area of the eye, Ref(217).
Titanium dioxide	May also be used in cosmetics intended for use in the area of the eye, Ref(217).
Ultramarine blue	External use only. May also be used in cosmetics intended for use in the area of the eye, Ref(217).
Ultramarines (green)	External use only. May also be used in cosmetics intended for use in the area of the eye, Ref(217).
Ultramarines (pink)	No reports on adverse effects.

Colorant	Remarks
Ultramarines (red)	No reports on adverse effects.
Ultramarines (violet)	No reports on adverse effects.
Zinc oxide	May also be used in cosmetics intended for use in the area of the eye, Ref(217).

Appendix C Psychic Aromatherapy

A discussion of essential oils and fragrances would not be complete without mentioning the use of fragrant plants by ritualists and individuals practicing "magical aromatherapy." This is probably the oldest branch of medicine and was practiced by ancient cultures like the Egyptians, Greeks, Romans, Kelts, and American Indians. They have long known that scents can awaken psychic awareness, arouse sexual desire, and deepen spirituality.

Magical aromatherapy usually includes visualization of desired changes with certain essential oils — a prayer to deity while burning incense, or visualization of business success or loving relationship enhanced by a combination of fragrances. Aromatherapy can have a powerful effect on the psyche, which may be the least understood part of the human mind.

In Table C-1 you will find a compilation of the magical aromatherapeutic qualities of essential oils as they have come down to us through the ages. The magic is real — bring it into your life.

Table C-1 Essential Oils used in Psychic Aromatherapy

Essential Oil	Psychic and/or Magical Influence
anise oil (illicum verum)	psychic awareness
bay oil (laurus nobilis)	psychic awareness, purification
benzoin balm (styrax benzoin)	physical and magical awareness, conscious mind; purifier, stimulant, comforting (euphoric and uplifting), drive out evil spirits, stimulate chakras, comforts anxiety conditions, helps with psychic exhaustion
bergamot oil (citrus bergamia)	peace, happiness, restful sleep; antidepressant; uplifting; anxiety, depression
camphor oil (cinnamomum camphora)	sleep. meditation, peace
caraway oil (carum carvi)	purification, physical energy, love; tonic; mental fatigue, mental strain
cardamom oil (elletaria cardamom)	love, sex

Essential Oil	Psychic and/or Magical Influence
cedar oil (cedrus atlantica)	spirituality, self control; appeasing, sedative, elevating, grounding, opening; deep relaxation, anxiety, stress, psychic work, yoga, meditation, ritual
celery oil (apium graveolens)	psychic awareness
chamomile oil (anthemis nobilis)	sleep. meditation, sleep; appeasing, realization; anger, tantrum, hypersensitivity, personal growth
cistus oil (cistus ladaniferus)	stimulant, sedative (nervous), elevating, grounding, opening; third eye, crown chakra, psychic centers, insomnia, nervousness, psychic work, meditation, rituals
coriander oil (coriandrum sativum)	memory, love healing
cypress oil (cupressus sempervirens)	easing loss, healing
eucalyptus oil (eucalyptus globulus)	health, purification, healing
fennel oil (foeniculum vulgare)	longevity, courage, purification
fir oil (abies sibirica, alba)	healing, purification, protection, physical energy, magical energy, money; elevating, grounding, opening; psychic work, third eye, crown chakra, anxiety stress, yoga, meditation, ritual
frankincense oil (boswellia carterii)	spirituality, meditation; fortifying, stimulant; mind, psychic centers, third eye, crown centers
geranium oil (pelargonium graveolens)	happiness, protection; stimulant, uplifting; depression, nervous tension
ginger oil (zingiber officinale)	magical energy, physical energy, love, sex, money, courage; stimulant; poor memory
honeysuckle oil (lonicera caprifolium)	weight loss, psychic awareness, prosperity
hyssop oil (hysoppus officinalis)	purification, conscious mind

Essential Oil	Psychic and/or Magical Influence
jasmine absolute (jasminum officinale)	love, peace, spirituality, sex, sleep. psychic dreams; stimulant, antidepressant, euphoric, uplifting; sexual chakra, anxiety, lethargy, menopause, sadness, lack of confidence, postnatal depression
juniper oil (juniperus communis)	protection, purification, healing; tonic; nervous and intellectual fatigue, poor memory
lavender oil (lavendula officinalis)	health, love, celibacy, peace, conscious mind; appeasing, antidepressant, calming, anticonvulsive; astral body, depression, convulsions
lemon oil (citrus limomum)	health, healing, physical energy, purification; antidepressant, uplifting; anxiety, depression
lemon balm oil (melissa officinalis)	peace, money purification; appeasing, antidepressant, calming, stimulant; astral body, depression, heart chakra, emotional shock, grief
lime oil (citrus aurantifolia)	purification, physical energy, purification; antidepressant, uplifting; anxiety, depression
mandarin oil	purification, joy, physical energy, magical energy; sedative; hysteria, insomnia, nervous tension
mugwort oil (artemisia vulgaris)	opening; dreams, psychic work
myrrh oil (commiphora myrrha)	love; fortifying, stimulant; mind, psychic centers, third eye, crown chakra
neroli oil (citrus vulgaris)	sedative, antidepressant, stimulant; hysteria, insomnia, emotional shock, grief, heart chakra
niaouli oil (melaleuca viridiflora)	protection, healing
nutmeg oil (myristica fragrans)	psychic awareness; stimulant; nervous and intellectual fatigue
orange oil (citrus aurantium)	purification, joy, physical energy, magical energy; sedative; hysteria, insomnia, nervous tension
palmarosa oil (cymbopogon martini)	love, healing
patchouli oil (pogostemon patchouli)	sex, physical energy, money; appeasing, antidepressant, calming; astral body, anxiety

Essential Oil	Psychic and/or Magical Influence
peppermint oil (mentha piperita)	conscious mind, purification; antidepressant, tonic, stimulant (nervous system); depression, fatigue, mental fatigue, mental strain
petitgrain oil (citrus aurantium)	conscious mind, protection; clarifying, refreshing, antidepressant, uplifting, tonic, stimulant; confusion, anxiety, depression, poor memory, mental fatigue, mental strain
pine oil (pinus sylvetris)	healing, purification, protection, physical energy, magical energy, money; appeasing, sedative; anxiety, stress
rose oil (rose damascena, rose centifolia)	love, peace, sex, beauty; stimulant, uplifting, antidepressant; heart chakra, emotional shock, grief, depression
rosemary oil (rosemarinus officinalis)	longevity, conscious mind, memory, love; appeasing, antidepressant, uplifting, tonic (nervous); astral body, depression, poor memory, mental fatigue, mental strain
sage oil (salvia officinalis)	euphoria, calm, dreams; antidepressant, uplifting, tonic (nervous); depression, exhaustion, mental fatigue
sandalwood oil (santalum album)	spirituality, meditation, sex, healing; elevating, grounding, opening, antidepressant, euphoric; third eye, crown chakra, yoga, meditation, rituals, depression
spearmint oil (mentha spicata)	healing, protection during sleep; antidepressant, tonic, stimulant (nervous system); depression, fatigue, mental fatigue, mental strain
spruce oil (-picea alba)	healing, purification, protection, physical energy, magical energy, money; elevating, grounding, opening; psychic work, third eye, crown chakra, yoga, meditation, rituals, anxiety, stress
vetiver oil (vetiveria zizanoides)	protection, money; stimulant, comforting; root chakra, ungroundedness
yarrow oil (achillea millefolium)	psychic awareness, courage, love

Essential Oil	Psychic and/or Magical Influence
ylang ylang oil (canagium odoratum)	peace, sex, love; antidepressant, euphoric, sedative, stimulant, calming; depression, menopause, stress, insomnia, nervous tension, sexual chakra, anger, frustration

References

1. Blount A.M., Geology Department, Amphibole (asbestos) content of cosmetic and pharmaceutical talcs, Rutgers University, Newark, NJ 07102, *Environ. Health Perspect.* 1991 Aug, 94, 225-30.

2. Kaji T., Kawashima T., Sakamoto M., Rhodamine B inhibition of glycosaminoglycan production by cultured human lip fibroblasts, Department of Environmental Science, Faculty of Pharmaceutical Sciences, Hokuriku University, Kanazawa, Japan, *Toxicol. Appl. Pharmacol.* 1991 Oct, 111(1), 82-9.

3. Reygagne A., Garnier R., Efthymiou M.L., Gervais P., [Glycerol monothioglycolate eczema in a hairdresser. Persistence of the allergen several weeks after the application of a permanent], Eczema au monothioglycolate de glycerol chez une coiffeuse. Persistance de l'allergene dans les cheveux plusieurs semaines apres l'application d'une permanente, Institut de Medecine du Travail, Hopital Fernand Widal, Paris, France. *J. Toxicol. Clin. Exp.* 1991 May-Jun, 11(3-4), 183-7.

4. Tosti A., Guerra L., Bardazzi F., Gasparri F., Euxyl K 400, a new sensitizer in cosmetics, Department of Dermatology, University of Bologna, Italy, *Contact Dermatitis.* 1991 Aug, 25(2), pp. 89-93.

5. Pigatto P.D., Bigardi A., Legori A., Altomare G.F., Carminati G., Allergic contact dermatitis from Tektamer 38 (dibromocyanobutane), 2nd Department of Dermatology, University of Milan, Italy, *Contact Dermatitis,* 1991 Aug, 25(2), pp. 138-9.

6. Zemtsov A., A case of contact allergy to Kathon CG in the United States, Department of Dermatology, Texas Tech University School of Medicine, Lubbock 79430, *Contact Dermatitis,* 1991 Aug, 25(2), 135.

7. Brandrup F., Nickel eyelid dermatitis from an eyelash curler, Department of Dermatology, Odense University Hospital, Denmark, *Contact Dermatitis.* 1991 Jul, 25(1), 77.

8. Ross J.S., White I.R., Eyelid dermatitis due to cocamidopropyl betaine in an eye make-up remover, St John's Dermatology Centre, St Thomas's Hospital, London, UK, *Contact Dermatitis.* 1991 Jul, 25(1), 64.

9. Jordaan H.F., Van-Niekerk D.J., Transepidermal elimination in exogenous ochronosis. A report of two cases, Department of Dermatology, University of Stellenbosch, Tygerberg, Republic of South Africa. *Am. J. Dermatopathol.*, 1991 Aug, 13(4), 418-24.

10. Babish J.G., Scarlett J.M., Voekler S.E., Gutenmann W.H., Lisk D.J., Urinary mutagens in cosmetologists and dental personnel, Department of Pharmacology, New York State College of Veterinary Medicine, Cornell University, Ithaca 14853-7401, *J. Toxicol. Environ. Health,* 1991 Oct, 34(2), 197-206.

11. Fisher A.A., Allergic cheilitis due to castor oil in lipsticks, New York University Medical School, *Cutis.*, 1991 Jun, 47(6), 389-90.

12. Goncalo S., Gil J., Goncalo M., Baptista A.P., Pigmented photoallergic contact dermatitis from musk ambrette, Coimbra, Portugal, *Contact Dermatitis.* 1991 Mar, 24(3), 229-31.

13. Romaguera C., Vilaplana J., Grimalt F., Hydroxybenzoic Acids adverse effects, Allergy Department of Dermatology, University and Hospital Clinic of Barcelona, Spain, *Contact Dermatitis,* 1991 Mar, 24(3), 224-5.

14. Losek J.D., Rock A.L., Boldt R.R., Cyanide poisoning from a cosmetic nail remover, Dept. of Pediatrics, Medical College of Wisconsin, Children's Hospital of Wisconsin, Milwaukee, *Pediatrics*, 1991 Aug, 88(2), 337-40.

15. Senff H., Kollner A., Tholen S., Frosch P.J., [Contact allergies to recently introduced preservatives (Kathon CG, benzisothiazolinone, Euxyl K 400, Biobans, Grotans, Bronopol, Germall II)] Kontaktallergien gegen neuere Konservierungsmittel, Klinik fur Dermatologie und Allergologie, St. Barbara-Hospital Duisburg, *Hautarzt*, 1991 Apr, 42(4), 215-9.

16. Eisenbrand G., Blankart M., Sommer H., Weber B., N-nitrosoalkanolamines in cosmetics, Department of Food Chemistry and Environmental Toxicology, University of Kaiserslautern, Germany, *IARC. Sci. Publ.*, 1991(105), 238-41.

17. Aberer W., Reiter E., [Contact eczema and epicutaneous tests--distribution of allergens and changes in the spectrum in Vienna (nickel 24%, cobalt 9%, chromates 6%, fragrances 16%, balsam of Peru 10%, Kathon 5%, neomycin 4%, parabens 3%, lanolin 2%, benzocaine 1%, thiuram-mix 2% and carba-mix 1%)], Kontaktekzem und Epikutantest--Allergenverteilung und Wandel des Spektrums in Wien, I. Universitats-Hautklinik, Wien, *Wien. Klin. Wochenschr.*, 1991, 103(9), 263-7.

18. Kamp E., Eisenbrand G., Long-chain N-nitroso-N-methylalkylamines in commercial cosmetics, light-duty dishwashing liquids and household cleaning preparations, Lebensmittelchemie und Umwelttoxikologie, Fachbereich Chemie, Universitat Kaiserslautern, Kaiserslautern, Germany, *Food Chem. Toxicol.*, 1991 Mar, 29(3), 203-9.

19. Averbeck D., Dardalhon M., Magana-Schwencke N., Repair of furocoumarin-plus-UVA-induced damage and mutagenic consequences in eukaryotic cells, Institut Curie-Section de Biologie, CNRS UA 1292, Paris, France, *J. Photochem. Photobiol. B.*, 1990 Jun, 6(1-2), 221-36.

20. Bluhm R., Branch R., Johnston P., Stein R., Aplastic anemia associated with canthaxanthin ingested for 'tanning' purposes, Department of Pharmacy, Vanderbilt University School of Medicine, Nashville, TN, *JAMA.* 1990 Sep 5, 264(9), 1141-2.

21. Dooms-Goossens A., Morren M., Dierickx C., Marien K., A patient bothered by unexpected sources of isothiazolinones, Department of Medical Research (Dermatology), Katholieke Universiteit Leuven, Belgium, *Contact Dermatitis*, 1990 Sep, 23(3), 192-3.

22. Waliszewski M., Szymczynski G.A., Determination of phthalate esters in human semen, Instituto de Medicina Forense Framboyanes, Fracc. Costa Verde, Veracruz, Mexico, *Andrologia.*, 1990 Jan-Feb, 22(1), 69-73.

23. Piriou-Robaglia A., Robaglia J.L., Bonerandi J.J., [Dermatitis from contact with perfume], Dermites de contact aux parfums, Service de Dermatologie, Hopital Ste Marguerite, Marseille, *Allerg. Immunol. Paris*, 1990 Sep, 22(7), 274-9.

23.a Barr R.D., McMaster University, The mercurial nephrotic syndrome, Hamilton, Ontario, Canada, *East Afr. Med. J.*, 1990 Jun, 67(6), 381-6.

24. Scalia S., Guarneri M., Menegatti E., Determination of 1,4-dioxane in cosmetic products by high-performance liquid chromatography, Department of Pharmaceutical Sciences, University of Ferrara, Italy, *Analyst*, 1990 Jul, 115(7), 929-31.

25. Dyall-Smith D.J., Scurry J.P., Mercury pigmentation and high mercury levels from the use of a cosmetic cream, Monash Medical Centre, Clayton, VIC, *Med. J. Aust.*, 1990 Oct 1, 153(7), 409-10, 414-5.

26. Tosti A., Guerra L., Morelli R., Bardazzi F., Prevalence and sources of sensitization to emulsifiers, a clinical study, Department of Dermatology, University of Bologna, Italy, *Contact Dermatitis*, 1990 Aug, 23(2), 68-72.

27. de-Groot A.C., Weyland J.W., Cosmetic allergy from the aminoketone colour basic blue 99 (CI

56059), Department of Dermatology, Carolus Hospital, Hertogenbosch, The Netherlands, *Contact Dermatitis*, 1990 Jul, 23(1), 56-7.

28. Tosti A., Piraccini B.M., Bardazzi F., Occupational contact dermatitis due to quaternium 15, Clinica Dermatologica, Bologna, Italy, *Contact Dermatitis*, 1990 Jul, 23(1), 41-2.

29. Westin J.B., Speigelhalder B., Preussmann R., Shani-J, Assay of suntan lotions for the carcinogenic, non-volatile N-nitrosamine N-nitrosodiethanolamine [published erratum appears in Cancer Lett 1990 Aug,53(1),79] -Department of Medical Ecology, School of Public Health, Hebrew University-Hadassah School of Medicine, Jerusalem, Israel, *Cancer Lett.*, 1990 Apr 20, 50(2), 157-60.

30. Matsukubo Y., [Cosmetic dermatitis. Its relationship with positive patch test results, clinical features and atopy], Department of Dermatology, Nippon Medical School, Tokyo, Japan, *Nippon. Ika. Daigaku. Zasshi*, 1990 Jun, 57(3), 276-84

31. Reinberg A., Koulbanis C., Soudant E., Nicolai A., Mechkouri-M, Smolensky-M, Day-night differences in effects of cosmetic treatments on facial skin. Effects on facial skin appearance. CNRS UA 581 (Chronobiologie-Chronopharmacologie) et Fondation Adolphe de Rothschild, Paris, France, *Chronobiol. Int.*, 1990, 7(1), 69-79.

32. Fisher A.A., Adverse nail reactions and paresthesia from "photobonded acrylate 'sculptured' nails", New York University Medical School, New York, *Cutis.*, 1990 May, 45(5), 293-4

33. Foussereau J., An epidemiological study of contact allergy to 5-chloro-3-methyl isothiazolone/3-methyl isothiazolone in Strasbourg, Clinique Dermatologique, Hopital Civil, Strasbourg, France, *Contact Dermatitis*, 1990 Feb, 22(2), 68-70.

34. Tosti A., Restani S., Lanzarini M., Contact sensitization to diazolidinyl urea, report of 3 cases, Clinica Dermatologica, Universita di Bologna, Italy, *Contact Dermatitis*, 1990 Feb, 22(2), 127-8.

35. Frosch P.J., White IR, Rycroft-RJ, Lahti-A, Burrows-D, Camarasa-JG, Ducombs-G, Wilkinson-JD, Contact allergy to Bronopol, Department of Dermatology, University of Heidelberg, FRG, *Contact Dermatitis*, 1990 Jan, 22(1), 24-6.

36. Richards R.N., Uy-M, Meharg G., Temporary hair removal in patients with hirsutism, a clinical study, Department of Medicine (Dermatology), North York General Hospital, University of Toronto, Ontario, Canada, *Cutis.*, 1990 Mar, 45(3), 199-202.

37. Kanta J., Hudec V., Barta R., Velebny V., Elastin powder produced for cosmetic purposes does not affect formation of granulation tissue, Sb. Ved. Pr. Lek. Fak. Karlovy Univerzity Hradci, Kralove, 1989, 32(4), 403-6.

38. Piekacz H., Kiss E., [Analysis of formaldehyde in various chemical products for household use and in shampoos and bath liquids], Oznaczanie formaldehydu w niektorych wyrobach chemii gospodarczej oraz badanie, jego obecnosci w szamponach i plynach kapielowych, *Rocz. Panstw. Zakl. Hig.*, 1989, 40(3), 235-9.

39. Dooms-Goossens A., Vandaele M., Bedert R., Marien K., Hexamidine isethionate, a sensitizer in topical pharmaceutical products and cosmetics, Department of Medical Research (Dermatology), University Hospital, Leuven, Belgium, *Contact Dermatitis*, 1989 Oct 21(4), 270.

40. Serrano G., Pujol C., Cuadra J., Gallo S., Aliaga A., Riehl's melanosis, pigmented contact dermatitis caused by fragrances, Department of Dermatology, General Hospital, Valencia, Spain, *J. Am. Acad. Dermatol.*, 1989 Nov, 21(5 Pt 2), 1057-60.

41. Kinnunen T., Hannuksela M., Skin reactions to hexylene glycol, Department of Dermatology, University of Oulu, Finland, *Contact Dermatitis*, 1989 Sep, 21(3), 154-8.

42. Hasen B.M., Berger M., The sensitizing capacity of coumarins (III), Department of Dermatology,

University Hospital, Hamburg, FRG, *Contact Dermatitis*, 1989 Sep, 21(3), 141-7.

43. Richfield-Fratz N., Baczynskyj W.M., Miller G.C., Bailey J.E. Jr, Isolation, characterization and determination of trace organic impurities in FD&C red no. 40, Division of Colors and Cosmetics, Food and Drug Administration, Washington, DC 20204, *J. Chromatogr.*, 1989 Apr 21, 467(1), 167-76.

44. Garioch J.J., Forsyth A., Allergic contact dermatitis from 4-isopropyl-dibenzoylmethane in a light moisturising cream, Dermatitis Investigation Unit, Belvidere Hospital, Glasgow, Scotland, *Contact Dermatitis*, 1989 Apr, 20(4), 312-3

45. de-Groot A.C., Oleamidopropyl dimethylamine, Department of Dermatology, Carolus and Willem-Alexander Hospital, s-Hertogenbosch (The Netherlands), *Derm. Beruf. Umwelt.*, 1989 May-Jun, 37(3), 101-5.

46. Perret C.M., Happle R., Contact sensitivity to diazolidinyl urea (Germall II), Department of Dermatology, University of Nijmegen, The Netherlands, *Arch. Dermatol. Res.*, 1989, 281(1), 57-9.

47. Senff H., Exner M., Gortz J., Goos M., [Contact allergy to a new preservative], Kontaktallergie auf einen neuen Konservierungsstoff, Universitats-Hautklinik Essen, *Derm. Beruf. Umwelt.*, 1989 Mar-Apr, 37(2), 45-6.

48. de-Groot A.C., Weyland J.W, Cosmetic allergy to the UV-absorber bornelone, Department of Dermatology, Carolus and Willem-Alexander-Hospital, The Netherlands, *Derm. Beruf. Umwelt.*, 1989 Jan-Feb, 37(1), 13-5.

49. Wilson A.G., White I.R., Kirby J.D., Allergic contact dermatitis from propyl gallate in a lip balm, St Bartholomew's Hospital, West Smithfield, London, England, *Contact Dermatitis*, 1989 Feb, 20(2), 145-6.

50. de-Groot A.C., Herxheimer A., Isothiazolinone preservative, cause of a continuing epidemic of cosmetic dermatitis, CM, Comment in, Lancet 1989 Apr 22,1(8643),910, Department of Dermatology, Carolus & Willem-Alexander Hospital, MD's-Hertogenbosch, Netherlands, *Lancet.*, 1989 Feb 11, 1(8633), 314-6.

51. Ligthelm A.J., Butow K.W., Weber A., Silica granuloma of a lymph node, Department of Oral Pathology, University of Pretoria, South Africa, *Int. J. Oral Maxillofac. Surg.*, 1988 Dec, 17(6), 352-3.

52. Caravati E.M., Litovitz T.L., Pediatric cyanide intoxication and death from an acetonitrile-containing cosmetic, Division of Emergency Medicine, University of Utah, Salt Lake City, *JAMA*, 1988 Dec 16, 260(23), 3470-3.

53. Branca M., Garcovich A., Linfante L.D., Macri A., Mantovani A., Olivetti G., Salvatore G., Macro- and microscopic alterations in 2 rabbit skin regions following topically repeated applications of benzoic acid n-alkyl esters, Istituto Superiore di Sanita, Universita Cattolica del S. Cuore, Roma, Italy, *Contact Dermatitis*, 1988 Nov, 19(5), 320-34.

54. Fisher A.A., Allergic contact dermatitis due to rosin (colophony) in eyeshadow and mascara, New York University Medical School, *Cutis.*, 1988 Dec, 42(6), 507-8.

55. Jones S.K., Kennedy C.T., Contact dermatitis from triethanolamine in E45 cream, Department of Dermatology, Bristol Royal Infirmary, UK, *Contact Dermatitis*, 1988 Sep, 19(3), 230.

56. Menne T., Hjorth N., Routine patch testing with paraben esters, Department of Dermatology, Gentofte Hospital, Hellerup, Denmark, *Contact Dermatitis*, 1988 Sep, 19(3), 189-91.

57. Hopkins M.P., Androff L., Benninghoff A.S., Ginseng face cream and unexplained vaginal bleeding, Department of Obstetrics and Gynecology, University of Michigan Medical Center, Ann Arbor 48109, *Am. J. Obstet. Gynecol.*, 1988 Nov, 159(5), 1121-2.

58. de-Groot A.C., van-der-Meeren H.L., Weyland J.W., Cosmetic allergy from stearic acid and glyceryl stearate, Department of Dermatology, Carolus & Willem-Alexander Hospital,

's-Hertogenbosch, The Netherlands, *Contact Dermatitis*, 1988 Jul, 19(1), 77-8.

59.   de-Groot A.C, Bruynzeel D.P., van-Joost T., Weyland J.W., Cosmetic allergy from myristyl alcohol, Department of Dermatology, Carolus & Willem-Alexander Hospital, 's-Hertogenbosch, The Netherlands. *Contact Dermatitis*, 1988 Jul, 19(1), 76-7.

60.   de-Wit F.S., de-Groot A.C., Weyland J.W., Bos J.D., An outbreak of contact dermatitis from toluenesulfonamide formaldehyde resin in a nail hardener, Department of Dermatology, University of Amsterdam, The Netherlands, *Contact Dermatitis*, 1988 May, 18(5), 280-3.

61.   Dooms-Goossens A., Debusschere K., Gladys K., Degreef H., Contact allergy to an emulsifier in a cosmetic lotion, Department of Medical Research (Dermatology), University Hospital, Katholieke Universiteit Leuven, Belgium, *Contact Dermatitis*, 1988 Apr, 18(4), 249-50.

62.   de-Groot A.C., van-Joost T., Bos J.D., van-der-Meeren H.L., Weyland J.W., Patch test reactivity to DMDM hydantoin. Relationship to formaldehyde allergy, Department of Dermatology, Carolus & Willem-Alexander Hospital, Hertogenbosch, The Netherlands, *Contact Dermatitis*, 1988 Apr, 18(4), 197-201.

63.   Rogers C.G., Boyes B.G., Matula T.I., Heroux-Metcalf C., Clayson D.B., A multiple end-point approach to evaluation of cytotoxicity and genotoxicity of erythrosine (FD and C Red No. 3) in a V79 hepatocyte-mediated mutation assay, Toxicology Research Division, Food Directorate, Health and Welfare Canada, Ottawa, Ont, *Mutat. Res.*, 1988 May-Aug, 205(1-4), 415-23.

64.   Dooms-Goossens A., de-Boulle K., Dooms M., Degreef H., Imidazolidinyl urea dermatitis, *Contact Dermatitis*, 1986 May, 14(5), 322-4.

65.   Ford G.P., Beck M.H., Reactions to Quaternium 15, Bronopol and Germall 115 in a standard series, *Contact Dermatitis*, 1986 May, 14(5), 271-4.

66.   Lowe N.J., Cutaneous phototoxicity reactions, *Br. J. Dermatol.*, 1986 Aug, 115 Suppl 31, 86-92.

67.   Hausen B.M., [Laurel allergy. Cause, effect and sequelae of the external application of a so-called nature remedy], Lorbeer-Allergie. Ursache, Wirkung und Folgen der ausserlichen Anwendung eines sogenannten Naturheilmittels, *Dtsch. Med. Wochenschr.*, 1985 Apr 19, 110(16), 634-8.

68.   Allyl isovalerate adverse effect, IARC Monogr. Eval. Carcinog. Risk Chem. Hum. 1985 Feb, 36, 69-74.

69.   English J.S., White I.R., Dermatitis from D & C Red No. 36, *Contact Dermatitis*, 1985 Nov, 13(5), 335.

70.   Goitre M., Bedello P.G., Cane D., Roncarolo G., Contact dermatitis from novocaine in Gerovital cream, *Contact Dermatitis*, 1985 Apr, 12(4), 234-5.

71.   Koch S.E., Mathias T., Maibach H.I., Chloracetamide, an unusual cause of cosmetic dermatitis [letter], *Arch. Dermatol.*, 1985 Feb, 121(2), 172-3.

72.   Valentino A., Fimiani M., Baiocchi R., Bilenchi R., Perotti R., Castelli A., Mancianti M.L., Raffaelli M., -[Cosmetic acne and a test of comedogenicity (cacao and linseed) oil], Acne cosmetica e test di comedogenicita', *Boll. Soc. Ital. Biol. Sper.*, 1984 Oct 30, 60(10), 1845-8.

73.   de-Groot A.G., Liem D.H., Contact allergy to oleamidopropyl dimethylamine, *Contact Dermatitis*, 1984 Nov, 11(5), 298-301.

77.   Spiegelhalder B., Preussmann R., Contamination of toiletries and cosmetic products with volatile and nonvolatile N-nitroso carcinogens, *J. Cancer Res. Clin. Oncol.*, 1984, 108(1), 160-3.

78.   Dooms-Goossens A., Vandekerckhove M., Verschave H., Degreef H., Cosmetic dermatitis due to methyl glucose sesquisterarate, *Contact Dermatitis*, 1984 May, 10(5), 312-3.

79.   Rantuccio F., Sinisi D., Coviello C., Conte A., Scardigno A., Histological changes in rabbits after application of medicaments and cosmetic bases (III), *Contact Dermatitis*, 1984 Apr, 10(4), 212-9.

80.   van-Joost T., Liem D.H., Stolz E., Allergic contact dermatitis to monotertiary-butylhydroquinone in lipgloss, *Contact Dermatitis*, 1984 Mar, 10(3), 189-90.

81.   Taylor J.S., Jordan W.P., Maibach H.I., Allergic contact dermatitis from stearamidoethyl diethylamine phosphate, a cosmetic emulsifier, *Contact Dermatitis*, 1984 Feb, 10(2), 74-6.

82.   Fulton J.E. Jr., Pay S.R., Fulton J.E., Comedogenicity of current therapeutic products, cosmetics, and ingredients in the rabbit ear (isopropyl myristate and its analogs, such as isopropyl palmitate, isopropyl isostearate, butyl stearate, isostearyl neopentanoate, myristyl myristate, decyl oleate, octyl stearate, octyl palmitate or isocetyl stearate. Propylene glycol-2 (PPG-2) myristyl propionate and lanolins), 3d, *J. Am. Acad. Dermatol.*, 1984 Jan, 10(1), 96-105.

83.   Bjorkner B., Niklasson B., Contact allergic reaction to D & C Yellow No. 11 and Quinoline Yellow, *Contact Dermatitis*, 1983 Jul, 9(4), 263-8.

84.   Fiedler H.P., [Formaldehyde and formaldehyde releasers], Formaldehyd -Formaldehyd-Abspalter, *Derm. Beruf. Umwelt*, 1983, 31(6), 187-9.

85.   Sai S., Lipstick dermatitis caused by ricinoleic acid, *Contact Dermatitis*, 1983 Nov, 9(6), 524.

86.   de-Groot A.C., Liem D.H., Facial psoriasis caused by contact allergy to linalool and hydroxycitronellal in an after-shave, *Contact Dermatitis*, 1983 May, 9(3), 230-2.

87.   Lavrijsen A.P., Vermeer B.J., Cosmetics and drugs. Is there a need for a third group, cosmeceutics? Department of Dermatology, University Hospital, Leiden, The Netherlands, *Br. J. Dermatol.*, 1991 May, 124(5), 503-4.

88.   Storrs F.J., Bell D.E., Allergic contact dermatitis to 2-bromo-2-nitropropane-1,3-diol in a hydrophilic ointment, *J. Am. Acad. Dermatol.*, 1983 Feb, 8(2), 157-70.

89.   Meynadier J.M., Meynadier J., Colmas A., Castelain P.Y., Ducombs G., Chabeau G., Lacroix M., Martin P., Ngangu Z., [Allergy to preservatives (formaldehyde (4.7 p. 100), Bronopol (4.7 p. 100), ammoniated mercury chloride (3.8 p. 100), benzoic acid (2.1 p. 100), sodium benzoate (1.9 p. 100), parabens (1.9 p. 100), dichlorophen (1.7 p. 100), chloracetamid (1.5 p. 100), benzyl benzoate (1.5 p. 100), Germall 115 (1.2 p. 100), butylhydroxyanisol (1 p. 100) and Dowicil (0.8 p. 100)], Allergie aux conservateurs, *Ann. Dermatol. Venereol.*, 1982, 109(12), 1017-23.

90.   Andersen K.E., [Skin irritation caused by propylene glycols], Hautreizungen durch Propylenglykol, Storrs-FJ *Hautarzt.*, 1982 Jan, 33(1), 12-4.

91.   Dybing E., Saxholm H.J., Aune T., Wirth P.J., Thorgeirsson S.S., Studies on mutagenic and carcinogenic N-substituted aryl compounds (aromatic diamines used in hair dyes), cosmetics and drugs, *Natl. Cancer Inst. Monogr.*, 1981 Dec(58), 21-26.

92.   Calnan C.D, Quinazoline yellow dermatitis (D & C Yellow 11) in an eye cream, *Contact Dermatitis*, 1981 Sep, 7(5), 271.

93.   Marzulli F.N., Anjo D.M., Maibach H.I., In vivo skin penetration studies of 2,4-toluenediamine, 2,4-diaminoanisole, 2-nitro-p-phenylenediamine, p-dioxane and N-nitrosodiethanolamine in cosmetics, *Food. Cosmet. Toxicol.*, 1981 Dec, 19(6), 743-7.

94.   Calnan C.D., Monotertiary butyl hydroquinone in lipstick, Contact-Dermatitis, 1981 Sep, 7(5), 280

95.   Monarca S., Fagioli F., Morozzi G., Evaluation of the potential carcinogenicity of paraffins for medicinal and cosmetic uses--determination of polycyclic aromatic hydrocarbons, *Sci. Total*

Environ., 1981 Jan, 17(1), 83-93.

96. Aune T., Nelson S.D., Dybing E., Mutagenicity and irreversible binding of the hepatocarcinogen, 2,4-diaminotoluene, *Chem. Biol. Interact.*, 1979 Apr, 25(1), 23-33.

97. Swift D.L., Zuskin E., Bouhuys A., Respiratory deposition of hair spray aerosol and acute lung function changes, *Lung.*, 1979, 156(2), 149-58.

98. Spencer P.S., Sterman A.B., Horoupian D.S., Foulds M.M., Neurotoxic fragrance produces ceroid and myelin disease (Acetyl ethyl tetramethyl tetralin (AETT)), *Science*, 1979 May 11, 204(4393), 633-5.

99. Marks J.G. Jr., Bishop M.E., Willis W.F., Allergic contact dermatitis to sculptured nails, *Arch. Dermatol.*, 1979 Jan, 115(1), 100.

100. Blondeel A., Oleffe J., Achten G., Contact allergy in 330 dermatological patients, *Contact Dermatitis*, 1978 Oct, 4(5), 270-6.

101. Palmer K.A., Denunzio A., Green S., The mutagenic assay of some hair dye components, using the thymidine kinase locus of L5178Y mouse lymphoma cells (m-phenylenediamine, 2 nitro-p-phenylenediamine, and 4-nitro-o-phenylenediamine, 2,4-diaminoanisole), *J. Environ. Pathol. Toxicol.*, 1978 Sep-Oct, 1(1), 87-91.

102. Hardel P.J., Reybet-Degat O., Jeannin L., Paqueron M.J., –[Hairdresser's asthma, hazards of hair bleaching agents containing alkaline persulphates (letter)], Asthme des coiffeurs, danger des decolorants capillaires contenant des persulfates alcalins, *Nouv. Presse. Med.*, 1978 Dec, 7(45), 4151.

103. Calnan C.D., Stinging sensation from ethoxyethyl--methoxy cinnamate, *Contact Dermatitis*, 1978 Oct, 4(5), 294, ISSN, 0105-1873.

104. Hoffman T.E., Adams R.M., Contact dermatitis to benzoin in greasepaint makeup, *Contact Dermatitis*, 1978 Dec, 4(6), 379-80.

105. Noster U., Hausen B.M., [Occupational dermatitis due to a yellow quinophthalone dye (solvent yellow 33, C.I. 47 000)], Berufsbedingtes Kontaktekzem durch gelben Chinophthalonfarbstoff (Solvent Yellow 33, C.I. 47 000), *Hautarzt.*, 1978 Mar, 29(3), 153-7.

106. Fahmy M.J., Fahmy O.G., Mutagenicity of hair dye components relative to the carcinogen benzidine in Drosophila melanogaster, *Mutat. Res.*, 1977 Sep, 56(1), 31-8.

107. Blijleven W.G., Mutagenicity of four hair dyes in Drosophila melanogaster (p-phenylenediamine, 2,4-diaminoanisole sulfate, 2,4-diaminotoluene and 4-nitro-0-phenylenediamine), *Mutat. Res.*, 1977 Apr, 48(2), 181-5.

108. Griesemer, Richard, Testimony by the National Cancer Institute before the Subcommittee on Oversight and Investigations of the House Committee on Interstate and Foreign Commerce on the Need for Cosmetic Safety Legislation, July 19, 1979.

109. Nissen S.H., Nielsen P.G., Unilateral mydriasis after use of propantheline bromide in an antiperspirant [letter], *Lancet.*, 1977 Nov 26, 2(8048), 1134.

110. Fiedler H.P., [Urea , properties, effects, use], TO, Harnstoff, Eigenschaften - Wirkung - Verwendung, *Berufsdermatosen*, 1977 Apr, 25(2), 63-6.

111. Gowdy J.M., Hexachlorophene lesions in newborn infants, Ulsamer-AG, *Am. J. Dis. Child.*, 1976 Mar, 130(3), 247-50.

112. Kruger-G, Thomas D.J., Disturbed oxidative metabolism in organic brain syndrome caused by bismuth in skin creams, Weinhardt, F., Hoyer, S., *Lancet.*, 1976 Sep 4, 1(7984), 485-7.

113. Hu S., A contribution to our knowledge of Leonurus L.(relieve from itches and shingles), i-mu-ts'ao, the Chinese motherwort, *Am. J. Chin. Med.*, 1976 Autumn, 4(3), 219-37.

114. Fisher A.A., Dooms-Goossens A., Persulfate hair bleach reactions. Cutaneous and respiratory

manifestations, *Arch. Dermatol.*, 1976 Oct, 112(10), 1407-9.

115.   Wright R.C., Allergic contact dermatitis from TEA-Coco hydrolyzed protein, Emmett-EA, *Arch. Dermatol.*, 1976 Jul, 112(7), 1008-9.

116.   National Institute for Occupational Safety and Health (NIOSH), *Pocket Guide to Chemical Hazards*, U.S. Department of Health and Human Services, June 1990.

117.   Pariser, R. J. (1977), Contact dermatitis to dioxybenzone. *Contact Dermatitis*, 3, 172.

118.   Fisher, Alexander A., M.D.(1978), *Contact Dermatitis*, Lea & Febinger, Philadelphia.

119.   Rudski, E. and Grzywa, Z. (1977), Dermatitis from arnica montana. *Contact Dermatitis*, 3, 281.

120.   Nater, Johan P., de Groot, Anton C., Liem, Dhiam H. (1983), Unwanted Effects of Cosmetics and Drugs in Dermatology, *Excerpta Medica*, Amsterdam Oxford Princeton.

121.   Afzelius, H. and Thukin, H. (1979), Allergic reactions to benzalkonium chloride, Contact Dermatitis, 5, 60.

122.   Lorenzetti, O.J. and Wernet, T.C. (1977), Topical parabens, benefit and risks, *Dermatologica* (Basel), 154,244.

123.   Maucher, O.M. (1974), Beitrag zur Kreuz oder Kopplungsallergie auf Parahydroxy benzoe saeure ester, *Berufsdermatosen*, 22, 183.

124.   North American Contact Dermatitis Group (1973), Epidemiology of contact dermatitis in North America, 1972, *Arch. Derm.*, 108, 573.

125.   Schorr, W.F. (1968), Paraben allergy. A cause of intractable dermatitis, *Amer. Med. Ass.*, 204, 859.

126.   Brown, R. (1979), Another case of sorbic acid sensitivity, *Contact Dermatitis*, 5, 268.

127.   Roed Petersen, J. and Hjorth, N. (1976), Contact dermatitis from anti oxydants, *Brit. J. Derm.*, 94, 233.

128.   Nakayama, H., Harada, R. and Toda, M. (1976), Pigmented cosmetic dermatitis, *Int. J. Derm.*, 15, 673.

129.   Hjorth, N. and Trolle Lassen, C. (1963), Skin reactions to ointment bases, *Trans. St. John's Hosp. derm. Soc. (London)*, 49, 127.

130.   Klingman, A.M. and Mills, O. H. (1972), Acne cosmetica. Arch. Derm., 106, 843.

131.   Maibach, H. I. (1978), Chronic dermatitis and hyperpigmentatioin from petrolatum, *Contact Dermatitis*, 4, 62.

132.   Sylvest, B., Hjorth, N. and Magnusson, B. (1975), Laurylether sulphate dermatitis, *Contact Dermatitis*, 1, 359.

133.   Petersen, H. O. (1977), Hypersensitivity to propolis. *Contact Dermatitis*, 3 278.

134.   Hannuksela, M., Kousa, M. and Pirilae, V. (1976), Contact sensitivity to emulsifiers, *Contact Dermatitis*, 2, 201.

135.   Fisher, A. A. (1974), Contact dermatitis from stearyl alcohol and propylene glycol, *Arch. Ferm.*, 110, 636.

136.   Hannuksela, M. (1979), Frequent contact allergy to higher fatty alcohols, *IV International Symposium on Contact Dermatitis*, San Francisco, March 29-31, 1979.

137.   Hannuksela, M. and Forstroem, L. (1976), Contact hypersensitivity to glycerol, *Contact Dermatitis*, 2, 105.

138.   Van Ketel, W. G. (1978), Contact dermatitis from ethanol, *Contact Dermatitis*, 1, 7.

139.   Rudzki, E. (1977), Contact urticaria from silk, *Contact Dermatitis*, 3, 53.

140.   Frost, Phillip, M.D., Horwitz, Steven N., *Principles of cosmetics for the dermatologist*, The C.V. Mosby Company, 1982.

141.   Treben, Maria, [Health from God's Pharmacy] *Gesundheit aus der Apotheke Gottes*, Verlag Wilhelm Ennsthaler, Steyr, Austria.

142.   Thompson, William A.R., *Medicines from the Earth*, McGraw Hill Book Company.

143.   Lukas Richard, *Nature's Medicines*, Parker Publishing Company, Inc., West Nyack, New York.

144.   Downing, J. G. (1951), Dangers involved in dyes, cosmetics, and permanent wave solutions applied to hair and scalp, *Arch. Derm.*, 63, 561.

145.   Rudzki, E. and Grzywa, Z., Dermatitis from arnica montana, *Contact Dermatitis*, 3, 281, 1977.

146.   Gerras, C. (1977), *The Complete Book of Vitamins*, Rodale Press, Emmaus, PA.

147.   Duke, James A., *CRC Handbook of Medicinal Herbs*, CRC Press, Inc., 1991.

148.   E. Steinegger, R. Haensel, *Lehrbuch der Pharmakognosie*, Springer, Berlin, 1972.

149.   Hawley, Gessner G., *The Condensed Chemical Dictionary*, New York, Van Nostrand Reinhold, 1987.

150.   U.S. Department of Health and Human Services, *Cosmetic Handbook*, U.S. Government Printing Office.

151.   Lautenschlager, H. Md., Roedinger J. Md, Ghyczy, M. Md., The Use of Liposomes from Soybean Phospholipids in Cosmetics, *SÖFW*, issue 14/88, p. 531-534.

152.   Nater, Johann P., De Groot, Anton C., Liem, Dhiam H., Unwanted effects of Cosmetics and Drugs used in Dermatology, *Excerpta Medica*, Amsterdam Oxford Princeton, 1983.

153.   Ames, Bruce N. Dr., Research on mutagenicity of hair dyes, Biochemistry Department of the University of California at Berkeley, 1978 Congressional Hearings.

154.   National Cancer Institute (National Toxicology Program), Carcinogenicity Results, Hair Dye and Cosmetic Ingredients and Related Chemicals, 1979 Congressional Hearings.

155.   Kaji T., Kawashima T., Yamamoto C., Sakamoto M., Rhodamine B inhibits collagen synthesis by human lip fibroblasts in culture, Department of Environmental Science, Faculty of Pharmaceutical Sciences, Hokuriku University, Kanazawa, Japan, *Toxicol. Lett.*, 1992 Jun, 61(1), 81-7.

156.   Martin R.F., Sanchez J.L., Gonzalez A., Lugo-Somolinos A., Ruiz H., Exogenous ochronosis, Department of Dermatology, School of Medicine, University of Puerto Rico, *P. R. Health Sci. J.*, 1992 Apr, 11(1), 23-6.

157.   Heindel J.J., Price C.J., Field E.A., Marr M.C., Myers C.B., Morrissey R.E., Schwetz B.A., Developmental toxicity of boric acid in mice and rats, Developmental and Reproductive Toxicology Group, National Institute of Environmental Health Sciences, Research Triangle Park, North Carolina 27709, *Fundam. Appl. Toxicol.*, 1992 Feb, 18(2), 266-77.

158.   Ross J.S., Cronin E., White I.R., Rycroft R.J., Contact dermatitis from Euxyl K 400 in cucumber eye gel, St. John's Dermatology Centre, St. Thomas's Hospital, London UK, *Contact Dermatitis*, 1992 Jan, 26(1), 60.

159.   Obara S., Muto H., Kokubo H., Ichikawa N., Kawanabe M., Tanaka O., Primary dermal and eye irritability tests of hydrophobically modified hydroxypropyl methylcellulose in rabbits, Specialty Chemicals Research Center, Shin-Etsu Chemical Co., Ltd., Niigata, Japan, *J. Toxicol. Sci.*, 1992 Feb, 17(1), 21-9.

160.   Reeve V.E., Mitchell L.E., Hazards of urocanic acid as a cosmetic ingredient, Department of Veterinary Pathology, University of Sydney, New South Wales, Australia, *Photodermatol. Photoimmunol. Photomed.*, 1991 Aug, 8(4), 176-80.

161.   Remaut K., Thune P., [Occurrence of cosmetic allergy] Hudavdelingen, Ulleval sykehus, Oslo, *Tidsskr. Nor. Laegeforen.*, 1992 Apr 10, 112(10), 1275-7.

162.   Scalia S., Menegatti E., Assay of 1,4-dioxane in commercial cosmetic products by HPLC, Dipartimento di Scienze Farmaceutiche, Universita di Ferrara, Italy, *Farmaco.*, 1991 Nov, 46(11), 1365-70.

163.   Morren M., Dooms-Goossens A., Heidbuchel M., Sente F., Damas M.C, Contact allergy to dihydroxyacetone, Department of Medical Research (Dermatology), University Hospital, Katholieke Universiteit Leuven, Belgium, *Contact Dermatitis*, 1991 Nov, 25(5), 326-7.

164.   Fischer T., Bergstrom K., Evaluation of customers' complaints about sunscreen cosmetics sold by the

Swedish pharmaceutical company, National Institute of Occupational Health, Solna, Sweden, *Contact Dermatitis*, 1991 Nov, 25(5), 319-22.

165. Hulsmans R.F., van-der-Kley A.M., Weyland J.W., de-Groot A.C., [Replacement of Kathon CG by Euxyl K 400 in cosmetics, from the frying pan into the fire?], Carolus Ziekenhuis, afd. Dermatologie, Hertogenbosch, *Ned. Tijdschr. Geneeskd.*, 1992 Mar 21, 136(12), 587-9.

166. de-Groot A.C., Bruynzeel D.P., Coenraads P.J., Crijns M.B., van-Ginkel C.J., van-Joost T., van-der-Kley J.J., Meinardi M.M., Smeenk G., Weyland J.W., Frequency of allergic reactions to methyldibromoglutaronitrile (1,2-dibromo-2,4-dicyanobutane) in The Netherlands, Department of Dermatology, Carolus Hospital, Hertogenbosch, The Netherlands, *Contact Dermatitis*, 1991 Oct, 25(4), 270-1.

167. Hayakawa R., Hirose O., Arima Y., Pigmented contact dermatitis due to musk moskene, Division of Dermatology, Nagoya University Branch Hospital, Japan, *J. Dermatol.*, 1991 Jul, 18(7), 420-4.

168. Hashimoto K., [Toxicology of acetonitrile], Department of Hygiene, School of Medicine, Kanazawa University, *Sangyo Igaku*, 1991 Nov, 33(6), 463-74.

169. Zhao B., Fan W.X., Facial contact dermatitis. Pathogenetic factors in China, Department of Dermatology, First Affiliated Hospital of Nanjing Medical College, People's Republic of China, *Int. J. Dermatol.*, 1991 Jul, 30(7), 485-6.

170. Nava C., Meneghini C.L., Sertoli A., Angelini G., Moroni P., Pierini F., Veneroni C., Farli M., Francalanci S., Gola M., [Contact dermatitis of the hands in housewives, preliminary data of a multicenter study], Istituto di Medicina del Lavoro-Universita di Milano, *G. Ital. Med. Lav.*, 1989 May-Jul, 11(3-4), 109-12.

171. Boucaud C., Latarjet J., [Burn by photosensitization during cosmetic use of methoxsalen (letter)], *Presse. Med.*, 1991 Nov 23, 20(39), 1945-6.

172. Karlberg A.T., Liden C., Ehrin E., Colophony in mascara as a cause of eyelid dermatitis. Chemical analyses and patch testing, Department of Occupational Dermatology, National Institute of Occupational Health, Stockholm, Sweden, *Acta. Derm. Venereol. Stockh.*, 1991, 71(5), 445-7.

173. Valnet, Jean, [Treatment of Illnesses with Plant Oils] *Treatment des Maladies par les essences des Plantes*, Maloine S.A., Editeur, Paris, 1986.

174. Keller, Erich, [Essences of Beauty] *Essenzen der Schoenheit*, Orbis Verlag fuer Publizistik GmbH, Munchen, Germany, 1992.

175. U.S. Department of Health and Human Services, *Registry of Toxic Effects of Chemical Substances*, DHHS (NIOSH) Publication No. 87 114 and CDROM supplements.

176. Reeve V.E., Mitchell L.E., Hazards of urocanic acid as a cosmetic ingredient. Department of Veterinary Pathology, University of Sydney, New South Wales, Australia, *Photodermatol. Photoimmunol. Photomed.*, 1991 Aug, 8(4), 176-80.

177. Fischer T., Bergstrom K., Evaluation of customers' complaints about sunscreen cosmetics sold by the Swedish pharmaceutical company. National Institute of Occupational Health, Solna, Sweden, *Contact Dermatitis*, 1991 Nov, 25(5), 319-22.

178. Hulsmans R.F., van-der-Kley A.M., Weyland J.W., de-Groot-A.C. [Replacement of Kathon CG by Euxyl K 400 in cosmetics, from the frying pan into the fire?] Vervangen van Kathon CG in cosmetica door Euxyl K 400, van de regen in de drup? Carolus Ziekenhuis, afd. Dermatologie, *Hertogenbosch. Ned. Tijdschr. Geneeskd.*, 1992 Mar 21, 136(12), 587-9.

179. Zhao B., Fan W.X., Facial contact dermatitis. Pathogenetic factors in China. Department of Dermatology, First Affiliated Hospital of Nanjing Medical College, People's Republic of China, *Int. J. Dermatol.*, 1991 Jul, 30(7), 485-6.

180. Scalia S., Menegatti E., Assay of 1,4-dioxane in commercial cosmetic products by HPLC. Dipartimento di Scienze Farmaceutiche, Universita di Ferrara, Italy, *Farmaco*, 1991 Nov, 46(11), 1365-70.

181. Pigatto P.D., Bigardi A., Legori A., Altomare G.F., Carminati G., Allergic contact dermatitis from Tektamer 38 (dibromocyanobutane), 2nd Department of Dermatology, University of Milan, Italy. *Contact Dermatitis*, 1991 Aug, 25(2), 138-9.

182. Zhao B., Fan W.X., Facial contact dermatitis. Pathogenetic factors in China, Department of Dermatology, First Affiliated Hospital of Nanjing Medical College, People's Republic of China, *Int. J. Dermatol.*, 1991 Jul, 30(7), 485-6.

183. Reygagne A., Garnier R., Efthymiou M.L., Gervais P., [Glycerol monothioglycolate eczema in a hairdresser. Persistence of the allergen in the hair several weeks after the application of a permanent] Eczema au monothioglycolate de glycerol chez une coiffeuse. Persistance de l'allergene dans les cheveux plusieurs semaines apres l'application d'une permanente. Institut de Medecine du Travail, Hopital Fernand Widal, Paris, France, *J. Toxicol. Clin. Exp.*, 1991 May-Jun, 11(3-4), 183-7.

184. Martin R.F., Sanchez J.L., Gonzalez A., Lugo-Somolinos A., Ruiz H., Exogenous ochronosis. Department of Dermatology, School of Medicine, University of Puerto Rico, *P. R. Health Sci. J.*, 1992 Apr, 11(1), 23-6.

185. Obara S., Muto H., Kokubo H., Ichikawa N., Kawanabe M., Tanaka O., Primary dermal and eye irritability tests of hydrophobically modified hydroxypropyl methylcellulose in rabbits. Specialty Chemicals Research Center, Shin-Etsu Chemical Co., Ltd., Niigata, Japan, *J. Toxicol. Sci.*, 1992 Feb, 17(1), 21-9.

186. Parry C., Eaton J., Kohl, a lead-hazardous eye makeup from the Third World to the First World, Graduate School of Public and International Affairs, University of Pittsburgh, PA, *Environ Health Perspect.*, 1991 Aug, 94, 121-3.

187. Boucaud C., Latarjet J., [Burn by photosensitization. During cosmetic use of methoxsalen (letter)] Brulure par photosensibilisation. Lors d'usage cosmetique de methoxalene, *Presse. Med.*, 1991 Nov 23, 20(39), 1945-6.

188. Hulsmans R.F., van der Kley A.M., Weyland J.W., de-Groot A.C., [Replacement of Kathon CG by Euxyl K 400 in cosmetics, from the frying pan into the fire?] Vervangen van Kathon CG in cosmetica door Euxyl K 400, van de regen in de drup? Carolus Ziekenhuis, afd. Dermatologie, *Hertogenbosch Ned. Tijdschr. Geneeskd.*, 1992 Mar 21, 136(12), 587-9.

189. Hayakawa R., Hirose O., Arima Y., Pigmented contact dermatitis due to musk moskene, Division of Dermatology, Nagoya University Branch Hospital, Japan, *J. Dermatol.*, 1991 Jul, 18(7), 420-4.

190. Fischer T., Bergstrom K., Evaluation of customers' complaints about sunscreen cosmetics sold by the Swedish pharmaceutical company. National Institute of Occupational Health, Solna, Sweden. *Contact Dermatitis*, 1991 Nov, 25(5), 319-22.

191. Guttormsen A.B., Husby P., Elsayed S., [Anaphylactic shock during elective cesarean section. Sensitizing mechanisms and follow-up] TO, Anafylaktisk sjokk under elektiv sectio caesarea. Utlosende mekanismer og oppfolging, *Tidsskr. Nor. Laegeforen.*, 1989 Nov 20, 109(32), 3321-3.

192. Baldo B.A., Harle D.G., Fisher M.M., In vitro diagnosis and studies on the mechanism(s) of anaphylactoid reactions to muscle relaxant drugs, *Ann. Fr. Anesth. Reanim.*, 1985, 4(2), 139-45.

193. Baldo B.A., Fisher M.M., Anaphylaxis to muscle relaxant drugs, cross-reactivity and molecular basis of binding of IgE antibodies detected by radioimmunoassay, *Mol. Immunol.*, 1983 Dec, 20(12), 1393-400.

194. Baldo B.A., Fisher M.M., Substituted ammonium ions as allergenic determinants in drug allergy, *Nature*, 1983 Nov 17-23, 306(5940), 262-4.

195. Yoshihira K., Kawasaki Y., Yamazaki T., Goda Y., Maitani T., In vitro effects of synthetic dyes on the syntheses of prostaglandin E2 (PGE2) and 5-hydroxyeicosatetraenoic acid (5-HETE), National Institute of Hygienic Sciences, Setagaya-ku, Japan, *J. Pharmacobiodyn.*, 1991 Jun, 14(6), 327-34.

196. Morren M., Dooms-Goossens A., Heidbuchel M., Sente F., Damas M.C., Contact allergy to dihydroxyacetone, Department of Medical Research (Dermatology), University Hospital, Katholieke Universiteit Leuven, Belgium, *Contact Dermatitis*, 1991 Nov, 25(5), 326-7.

197. Hannuksela M., Salo H., The repeated open application test (ROAT). *Contact Dermatitis*, 1986 Apr, 14(4), 221-7.

198. Eiermann H.J., Larsen W., Maibach H.I., Taylor J.S., Prospective study of cosmetic reactions, 1977-1980, North American Contact Dermatitis Group, *J. Am. Acad. Dermatol.*, 1982 May, 6(5), 909-17

199. Monarca S., Fagioli F., Morozzi G., Evaluation of the potential carcinogenicity of paraffins for medicinal and cosmetic uses--determination of polycyclic aromatic hydrocarbons, *Sci. Total. Environ.*, 1981 Jan, 17(1), 83-93.

200. Boyd A.S., An overview of the retinoids, Department of Dermatology, School of Medicine, Texas Tech University Health Sciences Center, Lubbock 79430, *Am. J. Med.*, 1989 May, 86(5), 568-74.

201. Bird D.F., Update on the effects of vitamins A, C, and E and selenium on carcinogenesis. Source (Bibliographic citation), *Proc. Soc. Exp. Biol. Med.*, 1986 Dec, 183(3), 311-20.

202. Lowe K.E., Norman A.W., Vitamin D and psoriasis, Department of Biochemistry, University of California, Riverside CA, *Nutr. Rev.*, 1992 May, 50(5), 138-42.

203. Salagnac V., Leonard F., de-Lacharriere O., Le-Corre Y., Kalis-B, Traitement du vieillissement actinique par la vitamine A acide topique a differentes concentrations [Treatment of actinic aging with topical vitamin A acid in different concentrations], Service de Dermatologie, Hopital Sebastopol, Reims, *Rev. Fr. Gynecol. Obstet.*, 1991 Jun, 86(6), 458-60.

204. Mock D.M., Skin manifestations of biotin deficiency, Department of Pediatrics, University of Iowa Hospitals and Clinics, Iowa City, *Semin. Dermatol.*, 1991 Dec, 10(4), 296-302.

205. Miller S.J., Nutritional deficiency and the skin, Division of Dermatology, University of California, San Diego School of Medicine, *J. Am. Acad. Dermatol.*, 1989 Jul, 21(1), 1-30.

206. Malone W.F., Studies evaluating antioxidants and beta-carotene as chemopreventives, Chemoprevention Branch, National Cancer Institute, Bethesda, MD, *Am. J. Clin. Nutr.*, 1991 Jan, 53(1 Suppl), 305S-313S.

207. Zamora-Martinez M.C., de-Pascual-Pola C.N., Medicinal plants used in some rural populations of Oaxaca, Puebla and Veracruz, Mexico, Centro de Investigaciones Forestales y Agropecuarias del Distrito Federal, INIFAP, Mexico, *J. Ethnopharmacol.*, 1992 Jan, 35(3), 229-57.

208. Werman M.J., Mokady S., Nimni M.E., Neeman I., The effect of various avocado oils on skin collagen metabolism, Department of Food Engineering and Biotechnology, Technion-Israel Institute of Technology, Haifa, Israel, *Connect. Tissue Res.*, 1991, 26(1-2), 1-10.

209. Bassett I.B., Pannowitz D.L., Barnetson R.S., A comparative study of tea-tree oil versus benzoylperoxide in the treatment of acne, Department of Dermatology, Royal Prince Alfred Hospital, Camperdown, NSW, *Med. J. Aust.*, 1990 Oct 15, 153(8), 455-8.

210. Perchellet J.P., Perchellet E.M., Belman S., Inhibition of DMBA-induced mouse skin tumorigenesis by garlic oil and inhibition of two tumor-promotion stages by garlic and onion oils, Division of Biology, Kansas State University, Manhattan 66506., *Nutr. Cancer*, 1990, 14(3-4), 183-93.

211. Rao A.R., Sadhana A.S., Goel H.C., Inhibition of skin tumors in DMBA-induced complete carcinogenesis system in mice by garlic (Allium sativum), Cancer Biology Laboratory, School of Life Sciences, Jawaharlal Nehru University, New Delhi, India, *Indian J. Exp. Biol.*, 1990 May, 28(5), 405-8.

212. Hegyi E., Suchy V., Nagy M., [Propolis allergy] Zur Frage der Propolisallergie, Lehrstuhl fur Dermatovenerologie der Medizinischen Fakultat, *Hautarzt*, 1990 Dec, 41(12), 675-9.

213. Krylova N.V., Besednova N.N., Solov'eva T.F., Loenko I.N., Faustov V.S., [Anti-inflammatory effect of polysaccharide obtained from ginseng cell cultures] Protivovospalitel'noe deistvie polisakharida, poluchennogo iz kul'tury kletok zhen'shenia, Konstantinova-NA, Smolina-TP, Eliakov-GB, *Antibiot. Khimioter.*, 1990 Apr, 35(4), 41-2.

214. Nishino H., Takayasu J., Iwashima A., Murakoshi M., Imanishi J., [Anticarcinogenesis activity of natural carotenes] Activite anticarcinogenetique des carotenes naturels, Departement de Biochimie, Universite Medicale de la Prefecture de Kyoto, *C. R. Seances. Soc. Biol. Fil.*, 1989, 183(1), 85-9.

215. Torresani C., Manara G.C., Bianchi M., De-Panfilis G., Trattamento della secchezza cutanea mediante l'impiego di un olio da bagno "fisiologico," *G. Ital. Dermatol. Venereol.*, 1989 Mar, 124(3), VII-XII.

216. Weber U., Goerz G., [Carotinoid retinopathy. III. Reversibility], Carotinoid-Retinopathie. III. Reversibilitat, *Klin. Monatsbl. Augenheilkd.*, 1986 Jan, 188(1), 20-2.

217. National Research Council, *Toxicity Testing: Strategies to Determine Needs and Priorities*, Washington, D.C., National Academy Press, 1984.

218. U.S. Department of Health and Human Services, *Federal Food, Drug, and Cosmetic Act, as Amended, and Related Laws*, Sec. 201(g)(1), Washington, D.C., 1989.

219. Proposed rule published by the U.S. Food and Drug Administration, "Sunscreen Drug Products for Over-the-Counter Human Use," 43 Fed. Reg. 38206, August 25, 1978.

220. Chen, J., An experimental study on the anti-senility effects of shou xing bu zhi, Chung. Hsi. I. Chieh. Ho. Tsa. Chi., 1989 Apr, 9 (4):226-7, 198.

Glossary

Acne A chronic skin disorder caused by inflammation of the hair follicles and the sebaceous glands. Acne spots are caused by overproduction of sebum and the obstruction and infection of the follicle. Acne can also be caused or fostered by certain cosmetic chemicals.

Allergic dermatitis Skin condition caused by the bodily immune system after skin is exposed to an antigen.

Alpha Hydroxy Acids Fruit acids used as biological ingredients for skin and hair care products as moisturizing and peeling agents.

Amphoteric surfactants Amphoteric surfactants are effective at all pH ranges. They become anionic in alkaline solutions, cationic at acid pH values and remain neutral or "zwitterionic" in neutral solutions.

Analgesic Substances that relieve pain. The two types of analgesic drugs are non narcotic and narcotic. Although most analgesics in use today are synthetic products, both types of analgesic occur naturally in plants.

Anodyne An agent that soothes and relieves pain. See analgesic.

Antiaging Substances and behavior that can prevent premature aging of the skin caused by environmental influences and nutritional deficiencies. However, the natural aging process of the body and skin cannot be altered by elixirs or drugs.

Antibacterial A group of substances that can kill bacteria and are used to treat infections. They are also used to preserve food and cosmetic products.

Antibiotic A group of complex organic substances used to treat infections caused by bacteria. Originally derived from molds and fungi, antibiotics are now made synthetically. There are some herbs that also have antibiotic qualities.

Anticarcinogen An agent that prevents the formation of carcinomas in the body or skin. It also includes substances that can arrest or heal skin cancers.

Anticellulite An agent that counteracts bacterial infection of skin tissues. It can also include substances that restore or strengthen the natural barrier of the skin to avoid bacterial infection. See cellulitis.

Antidandruff An agent that controls excessive formation of dandruff cells from the horny layer of the skin. It may also alleviate the itching and scaliness associated with seborrheic dermatitis. See dandruff.

Antidepressant In aromatherapy a combination of fragrances that can lift a feeling of sadness, hopelessness, and a general loss of interest in the environment.

Antigen A substance that can trigger an immune response, resulting in the production of antibodies as part of the body's immune system. Many of them are proteins not found in the human body, including microorganisms and toxins.

Antiinflammatory An agent that can soothe the redness, swelling, heat, and pain due to a chemical or physical injury, or infection. Also, property of a substance that can prevent inflammation and adverse effects due to toxic cosmetic ingredients.

Antiirritant An agent that counteracts localized, superficial inflammation of the skin that is due directly to one or more external substances.

Antimicrobial A popular term for an agent that protects tissues from invasion by microorganisms or aids in the preservation of food and cosmetic products. See antibacterial.

Antioxidants A group of substances that prevent the oxidation of fats and oil and the formation of free radicals in food, cosmetic products and in living tissues. Vitamin E is an example of a natural antioxidant.

Antiperspirant A product or agent that controls excessive sweating including the associated odor due to bacterial growth. Synthetic deodorants are rated high risk products because of side effects they can create.

Antiseborrheic A substance that controls the excessive secretion of sebum, and reduces oiliness of the face and greasy scalp, a condition that is most common in adolescent boys and some girls.

Antiseptic Substances applied to the skin to destroy bacteria and other microorganisms and prevent infections. See antibacterial.

Antiwrinkle Cosmetic product that prevents the premature formation of wrinkles in the face and around the eyes. Although the natural aging process cannot be stopped, much can be done to smooth existing conditions with deep moisturizers and proper nourishment of the skin cells.

Approved colorants A list of approved colorants issued by the U.S. Department of Health and Human Services. See also certified colors.

Aromatherapy A range of treatments using aromatic essential oils extracted from plants. The patient describes his or her symptoms to the therapist who chooses the most appropriate oil for massage or incorporation into creams, lotions, bath preparations, or inhalants.

Astringent A substance that causes tissues to dry and shrink by reducing their ability to absorb water. Astringents are widely used in antiperspirants and skin toners. They also can promote the healing of inflamed skin.

Bacteria A group of single cell microorganisms that can cause disease by producing poisons that are harmful to human cells. The undamaged skin has natural substances that prevent bacteria from entering living tissues. These substances can easily be depleted by synthetic cosmetic materials.

Carcinogen Any physical or chemical agent that causes or supports the development of cancer, like UV radiation or asbestos.

Cellulitis A bacterial infection of skin tissues. Affected are usually the face, neck, or legs where the skin feels hot, tender, and red. (The person is often feverish.)

Certified colors Colorants used in food, drugs, and cosmetics products that are approved by the FDA. Manufacturers of colorant materials are required to submit samples of production batches to the FDA for certification of purity before marketing.

CFR Code of Federal Regulations. The CFR has several laws that apply to the cosmetics and hair care industry. The main provisions of the law deal with Adulterated and Misbranded Cosmetics, Cosmetic Safety, and Cosmetic Labeling and Declaration of Ingredients.

Chelate Any chemical compound that is able to chemically bind heavy metal salts and make them insoluble in water. Heavy metal salts act as catalyst in cosmetic preparations and in the human body in breaking down unsaturated fatty acids and the formation of free radicals.

Cholesterol A lipoid manufactured by the liver from where it is distributed by the blood throughout the body. It mostly occurs in brain tissue, fatty tissues, and in the skin. It forms a natural protective skin cream with sebum and water to lubricate and protect the skin.

Coal tar colors Most synthetic colorant materials are called coal tar colors because many of the first synthetic colors were obtained from coal tar products. Today's raw materials are no longer derived from coal but from petro chemicals.

Comedogenic Promotes the formation of acne. See acne.

Contact dermatitis Skin reactions caused as a result of external contact with toxic substances.

Contaminants Many synthetic cosmetic raw materials are contaminated with manufacturing byproducts. These are potent toxins and many have carcinogenic and mutagenic properties. The most important ones are dioxane, ethylene oxide, nitrosamines, heavy metal compounds, and asbestos.

Cosmetics The CFR defines cosmetics as "articles intended to be applied to the human body for cleansing, beautifying, promoting attractiveness or altering the appearance without affecting the body's structure or function." Cosmetic products intended to affect the structure or functions of the human body (like antiwrinkle preparations) must meet the more stringent regulations intended for the drug industry. Most of drug-related ingredients contained in such cosmetic products are components of over-the-counter drugs.

CTFA The Cosmetics, Toiletry, and Fragrance Association. The CTFA represents over 90 percent of the manufacturers of cosmetic materials and products in the United States. It is powerful congressional lobby which has traditionally opposed tighter control of the cosmetic industry.

Cytotoxicity Attribute of a group of substances that kill or damage cells. Cytotoxins primarily affect abnormal and cancer cells, but they also can damage healthy cells.

Dandruff A common, harmless, but irritating condition in which dead cells of the horny layer of the scalp are shed, producing unsightly white flakes in the hair and on clothing. The usual cause of dandruff is seborrheic dermatitis that shows up as an itchy, scaly rash on the scalp.

Deodorant A substance that removes bad-smelling odor, especially body odors caused by the decomposition of sweat. Deodorants can contain antiseptic substances to destroy bacteria, and fragrances to mask the odor.

Deoxyribonucleic acid See DNA.

Dermatitis Inflammation of the skin. The main types of dermatitis are erythema, eczema, seborrhea, contact dermatitis, allergic dermatitis, and urticaria.

DNA Commonly used abbreviation for deoxyribonucleic acid. DNA is the principle carrier of genetic information in almost all organisms. Some chemical substances used in cosmetics can damage the genetic information and cause mutation, including cancer.

Eczema An inflammation of the skin, usually causing itching and sometimes accompanied by scaling and blistering. Eczema is sometimes caused by an allergy.

Emulsifier Surface active natural or synthetic compound that can simultaneously bind water and oil on a molecular level and form an emulsion.

Erythema Redness of the skin. It can be the initial state of contact dermatitis. Facial erythema can have many causes, including blushing, hot flashes, sunburn, dermatitis, eczema, and urticaria.

Essential fatty acids Fatty acids that cannot be synthesized in the human body. The most important ones are the linoleic, linolenic, and arachidonic acids. They are also called Vitamin F and are building blocks for a class of important regulating substances in the human body.

Essential oils Volatile and strong smelling botanical compounds of oil-like consistency that are insoluble in water but are readily soluble in alcohol or hydrocarbon solvents. Many plants have characteristic odors that are mostly pleasant. −They are a complicated mixture of organic chemicals whose importance lies in their use for perfumes and cosmetics, medicine, aromatherapy, as well as for spices and flavor materials in the food industry.

Expectorants A group of substances used to promote the coughing up of phlegm. Many plant materials, especially essential oils, have expectorant qualities and have been used for that purpose prior to the development of modern medicines.

FDA Food and Drug Administration. The U.S. Department of Health and Human Services, Food and Drug Administration (FDA) is responsible for regulating all matters related to food, drugs, and cosmetics.

Free radicals Short-lived, reactive chemical compounds that contain an unpaired electron. They react with constituents of a living cell thereby destroying the cell. They are believed to be one important factor in the natural aging process. Some free radicals are formed inside the body from unsaturated fatty acids and atmospheric pollutants like ozone. Vitamin E and other antioxidants have the ability to prevent the formation of free radicals inside the body.

Fungicidal An agent that kills fungal organisms that cause fungal infections of the skin. The most common fungal infections are athlete's foot and thrush.

Hair colors A group of coal tar colorants that is not regulated by the FDA as part of the 1938 Food, Drug and Cosmetic Act, the law that outlines the regulatory responsibility of the FDA. After several studies done by the National Cancer Institute and others, it is established that many hair dyes are either carcinogens or mutagens and pose a serious health threat to the consumer.

Hydrophilic Property of molecules or parts of molecules that show affinity to water.

Hygroscopic Property of substances or molecules that attract water from the surroundings. They are used in cosmetics as part of moisturizing ingredients in creams and lotions. Some are able to extract moisture from the surrounding skin and defeat the purpose of keeping the skin moist.

Hypersensitivity An overreaction of the immune system to an antigen. Hypersensitivity occurs only on second or subsequent exposures to a particular antigen. It can cause asthma, hay fever, urticaria, and other skin reactions.

Irritant dermatitis A term describing a localized, superficial inflammation of the skin that is due directly to one or more external substances. Repeated application of these substances may develop into full-fledged dermatitis.

Keratosis A skin growth caused by an overproduction of keratin. Solar keratosis can form small, wartlike, red- or flesh-colored growths that appear on exposed parts of the body as a result of overexposure to the sun over a prolonged period of time.

Lipophilic Property of substances or molecules that show affinity to oil or other fatty substances.

Liposomes Microscopic cell-like structures formed from phospholipids. Liposomes are able to penetrate the horny layer of the skin and carry substances to the cell level.

Mutagen Any physical or chemical agent that effects a change in the genetic material within a cell. They can give rise to cancer or hereditary disease.

Myeloma A malignant cancerous condition characterized by the uncontrollable proliferation of cells.

NIOSH National Institute for Occupational Safety and Health. NIOSH develops and periodically revises recommended exposure limits for hazardous substances or conditions in the work place, acting under the authority of the Occupational Safety and Health Act of 1970.

Permeability, Skin Care The openness of the skin layers to penetration and passage of natural and synthetic substances into the body.

pH The degree of acidity or alkalinity of a solution. A value of seven indicates a neutral state. Larger than seven indicates an alkaline solution, smaller than seven indicates an acidic solution.

Phototoxins A wide range of chemical substances, both synthetic and natural, that develop toxic derivatives when exposed to solar radiation. They are very harmful to the skin and must be avoided.

Preservative An agent that prevents spoilage in food and cosmetic preparations by microorganisms or oxidation. Almost all preservatives have been shown to produce adverse effects in humans. The argument for their continued use is that the benefits of using preservatives outweigh the risk of deaths and injuries caused by spoiled food and cosmetics.

Psoriasis A common skin disease characterized by thickened patches of inflamed, red skin, often covered by silvery patches. It is caused when new skin cells are produced at about ten times the normal rate by the basal layer.

Psychic aromatherapy A range of treatments using aromatic essential oils extracted from plants similar to aromatherapy. The person seeking psychic experiences chooses the most appropriate oil for massage or incorporation into creams, lotions, bath preparations, or inhalation.

Ribonucleic acid See RNA

RNA Commonly used abbreviation for ribonucleic acid. RNA carries the inherited, coded instruction within a cell for proper cellular function. It works in conjunction with DNA to decode its instruction for the proper function of the human cell.

RTECS Registry of Toxic Effects of Chemical Substances. RTECS is published by NIOSH and registers more than 88,000 chemicals. Only a small number of these have been thoroughly studied and established as toxic. Many of today's cosmetic chemicals and contaminants are registered in RTECS and labeled as toxic.

Rubefacient A gentle local irritant that produces redness of the skin and increases micro circulation. Many essential oils have this property and are used as ingredients of massage oils.

Sarcoma Cancers of connective tissue. The cancer of the connective tissues in the skin is also called Kaposi's sarcoma.

Seborrhea Excessive secretion of sebum, causing increased oiliness of the face and a greasy scalp. This condition is most common in adolescent boys and some girls. It can lead to seborrheic dermatitis and acne conditions.

Sebum An oily secretion composed of oils and waxes and emulsifying substances, produced by the sebaceous glands in the skin. Sebum lubricates the skin and forms a natural skin cream with water.

SPF Solar Protection Factor. A measure of effectiveness of a sunscreen to protect against solar radiation. SPF lets you determine safe sun exposure time using a sunscreen, compared to safe exposure time without protection.

Sterolins Sterolins are plant steroids, also known as phyto sterolins. They are a subgroup of glycosides and are used in cosmetics because of their superior skin softening properties.

Surfactant Surfactants are surface active natural or synthetic compounds that are water soluble. They have both hydrophilic and lipophilic locations on the same molecule. This allows surfactants to attach to oils and bring them into solution similar to soaps.

Systemic effects Effect on the body as a whole. It is a term used in connection with determining the toxicity of topically applied creams and lotions on the entire body.

Thrush Infection of the mouth or genital regions by the fungus candida albicans.

Toxins Any number of substances that are dangerous to life and well-being. The long-term effect of small amounts of toxins in food, cosmetics and the environment are of particular interest. The population is at risk because a large number of potential toxins are contained in food and cosmetics and are used on a daily basis. There is no aggressive program by industry or government to improve this condition.

Tumorigenic An agent that causes tumors in humans and animals

Ultraviolet see UV

Urticaria A skin condition commonly known as hives, characterized by the development of raised white lumps surrounded by an area of red inflammation. The most common mechanism is an allergic reaction to external or internal sensitizers.

UV Ultraviolet Radiation. The invisible spectrum of solar radiation immediate beyond the violet of the visible light spectrum. It is divided into three regions with increasing danger to the skin; UV A, UV B, and UV C.

Vitamin Any group of complex chemicals that are essential for normal functioning of the body. With few exceptions (Vitamin D), the human body cannot manufacture these substances. They must be supplied through diet or by topical application to the skin.

Index